PENGUIN BOOKS

NOTHING MUCH HAPPENS

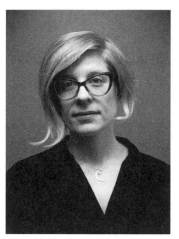

Photo by Megan Elise Crimmins-Helton

Kathryn Nicolai is the creator of the enormously successful podcast *Nothing Much Happens*. Nicolai is an architect of coziness, writing soothing stories that both ease the reader in to peaceful sleep and teach the principals of mindfulness, so that waking hours also become sweet and serene. She leans on her years of experience as a yoga and meditation teacher in order to seamlessly blend together storytelling and brain-training techniques that build better sleep habits over time. She is the owner of Ethos Yoga. She lives in Michigan with her wife and two dogs.

nothingmuchhappens.com

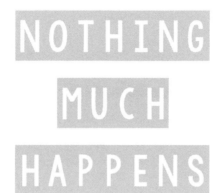

NOTHING MUCH HAPPENS

Cozy and Calming Stories

to Soothe Your Mind

and Help You Sleep

Kathryn Nicolai

ILLUSTRATIONS BY LÉA LE PIVERT

life

LIBRARY OF CONGRESS CATALOGING-IN-PUBLICATION DATA
Names: Nicolai, Kathryn, author.
Title: Nothing much happens : cozy and calming stories to soothe
your mind and help you sleep / Kathryn Nicolai.
Description: New York : Penguin Books, 2020. | Includes index.
Identifiers: LCCN 2020022797 (print) | LCCN 2020022798 (ebook) |
ISBN 9780143135913 (hardcover) | ISBN 9780525507499 (ebook)
Classification: LCC PR9199.4.N553 A6 2020 (print) |
LCC PR9199.4.N553 (ebook) | DDC 791.46/72—dc23
LC record available at https://lccn.loc.gov/2020022797
LC ebook record available at https://lccn.loc.gov/2020022798

Printed in the United States of America
1 3 5 7 9 10 8 6 4 2

BOOK DESIGN BY LUCIA BERNARD

For Jacqui, who makes my dreams come true

CONTENTS

How to Use This Book

. ' . ' ·

S leeping should be easy.

After all, it's one of the most natural things for us to do; we need rest and we want to sleep. But sometimes we just can't. What's going on there? Well, most times our brains get in the way. The thinking mind is a bit like a truck with a brick on the gas pedal. It keeps going even when no one is there to steer it, and it'll race all night if it's allowed to. Add to that racing mind a busy, chaotic world, too much caffeine, and a scary amount of screen time, and it becomes obvious why so many of us aren't finding sleep to be so easy.

But not to worry, friends; we can reclaim easy sleep and all the benefits and goodness that come along with it. It'll take a little practice and the discipline to set a routine in place, but I promise before long you'll be getting to sleep faster and staying asleep longer than you have since you were a kid. You'll wake up feeling rested and relaxed, and you might even find that these stories plant a few extra seeds of mindfulness in your waking life as well. (Bonus!)

Sleeping is a modern superpower.
Stories are old magic.

One of my earliest memories is of lying in bed and telling myself a story to fall asleep. I was probably four years old, and I still remember the story: a rags-to-riches tale with suspense and the sort of twists of fate that were part of the fairy tales my parents read to me. It had a happy, satisfying ending, and no matter how many times I told it, it worked to settle me before bed.

Whether I was using my own imagination to piece together a plot by moonlight or my parents sat on the edge of my bed reading someone else's tale, I naturally gravitated to the time-honored tradition of telling a story to prepare for sleep. The truth is, I've never stopped telling myself stories when I climb into bed at the end of each day. And though they've evolved to feature fewer pirate ships and dastardly villains and more simmering pots of soup and sleeping dogs, they still work just as well.

We tell stories before bed for a good reason. Stories help us make sense of things; they can point us in a useful direction and give us a way to step out of the present and into a new place and time. They offer new perspectives and new ways of imagining our lives—and the lives of others. And when they're told in a certain way, they can help us calm down.

I've been a full-time yoga teacher for seventeen years, and a regular meditator since 2003. In that time, I've learned a lot about how to trigger the body's relaxation response and how the principles of mindfulness—paying attention to what is happening moment to moment in a relaxed way—helps staticky minds to quiet. Along the way I've studied a bit of neuroscience, and my library, along with books about physiology and pranayama, is stocked with books about brains and how to train them.

One of the key things I learned was that neurons that fire together wire together, which means that good habits can be a matter of practice. I had certainly experienced that myself: I had trained my brain over the years with my lifelong practice of using stories to sleep, and now sleep and relaxation are an automatic response to supine storytelling.

But as I got older, I began to hear friends and family talking about their sleepless nights, anxiety, and chronic insomnia. I started to see just how debilitating those conditions can be, from increasing our risks for heart disease, depression, and anxiety to generally just feeling lousy and grouchy. I realized my storytelling practice was actually a secret superpower—one other people desperately needed. But barring literally being there with them as they tossed and turned (which is both creepy and impractical), I wasn't sure how to help.

One night I was (ironically) up in the middle of the night with my aging dog. As I sat with my beagle and rubbed her back, it hit me. A podcast with my stories. I could tuck people in at night with my voice. I could be there with my friends and family (and hopefully some other folks too) at bedtime. That night, sitting on the floor at three in the morning, I ordered a microphone.

Nothing Much Happens launched about six weeks later, and almost immediately I saw that my hunch was correct. I started to receive messages from listeners all over the world who told me that they were sleeping through the night for the first time in years or decades. This superpower was shareable.

I also began to hear about the other ways that listeners were using the stories. I heard about the man who listened while getting his chemotherapy, about the woman who'd been afraid to go to bed for years because of night terrors but now looked forward to tucking herself in at night and having pleasant dreams for almost the first time in her life. People wrote to say they had successfully gotten off sleep medications and that they felt rested and alert when their alarms went off in the morning. Families told me they listened together before bed and that little ones who'd been running around the house chicken-sans-head style had settled and slept within minutes. People listened when they felt anxious and then they felt better. Artists wrote to say they liked to listen while they drew or sculpted, and sometimes they'd send a picture of the art that the story had inspired.

This is the power of stories, and this is how I know that they work.

How to sleep.

One of the reasons we often struggle to shift from work mode into sleep mode is that we now carry work right into bed with us. We answer emails, obsessively check the same three or four social media apps, and receive and send texts moments before we try to find rest. No wonder the mind resists sleep or wakes us up at three in the morning to try to solve a problem we were working on just before we fell asleep. As far as our brains know we're still working. We need to close the loops on our day in order to signal to our minds that work is over for the time being.

To get into these better sleep habits, you're going to need to set some boundaries. If you can leave all your devices outside your bedroom, that's great. Really, that's ideal. It would change a lot. But if that's not going to happen for you, you'll need to draw a boundary somewhere else. Say thirty minutes before you want to start sleeping, you shut things down, switch your phone to do not disturb mode, and put everything with a screen in a drawer. Once work stuff is tucked away, undertake a little "Going to bed ritual." Rituals can be really helpful in shifting us from one mindset to another. Your ritual might include brushing your teeth, washing your face, laying out clothes for the morning, saying good night to your pets or family members, or fixing a late-night cup of herbal tea. The idea is that you are creating a routine that signals to your mind and body that it's almost bedtime, so you'll want to fill this time with the things that signal that to you.

Next, get into bed and get comfortable. Adjust everything until it feels just right and let your whole body relax into your sheets.

Now that you've stepped away from your waking life and started the countdown clock for sleep, you need to give your mind someplace to rest. That's where these stories come in. They are like a soft nest to lay your mind into, a cozy landing place after a busy day. Remember that truck with the brick on the gas pedal? Well, the stories are a tidy, well-organized garage to park it in. They're simple and nothing much happens in them and that's the idea.

As you read, let the details of the stories help you build a scene in your mind that you can really settle into. Lean into the parts that feel particularly cozy. Look at the illustrations and take in the specifics. When your eyes begin to droop, set down the book, turn off the light, and let your body be heavy and relaxed. Take a deep breath in through your nose and out through your mouth. Do it again. Breathe in and out. Good. You might even say to yourself, "I'm about to fall asleep, and I'll sleep deeply all night." As you lie drifting closer and closer to sleep, stay in the story by walking yourself though any of the details you can remember—especially anything that felt particularly cozy.

Sleep.

How to go back to sleep if you wake in the middle of the night.

Many people have no trouble at all falling asleep; it's staying asleep that they struggle with. Often in those predawn hours the mind is allowed to turn back on: the truck engine revs to life, and getting back to sleep can feel impossible. The key in those moments is to get your mind back into the nest as soon as possible.

To do that let's take one of our stories as an example. Imagine you're reading the story "A Block from Home," in which a person is heading home in the rain. See if you can put yourself in their position as they stop to buy pears and a small packet of almonds. Then, after they get home and turn the locks on the door to shut the world out, they lie on a sofa, and a kitty jumps up to join them. Doesn't that feel nice? Doesn't it feel just right?

Upon waking in the night, bring your mind right back to those details. I find it really helps to say the title of the story in your mind to signal to yourself that you are going into that world. Say to yourself, "A Block from Home." Then think about the pears and almonds. Think about how it feels to get home on a rainy night and close the door behind you. Imagine yourself moving through the rooms of your house or apartment, lying down on your sofa, and drifting off to sleep. Doing this will disrupt your brain's tendency to cycle through thoughts and worries. I promise. It will work.

When I started the podcast, along with all those emails from listeners saying the stories had put them to sleep, many more came from people who said that this particular technique worked for them as well as it always had for me. I saw reviews saying, "If I wake up in the middle of the night, I do what Kathryn says and think my way through the story and I go right back to sleep!"

This is brain training. Be patient. Be diligent. In time you will be amazed at how well you sleep. You will find yourself looking forward to bed, knowing that you have a sweet place to rest your mind till morning.

How to relax.

Besides sleeping you may find you need help being calm and staying centered during the day. First let me say, you are not alone. Many, many people struggle with anxiety. It is incredibly common, and when you combine the hair trigger on our fight-or-flight response with modern life, well, you'd be a rare person if you never felt anxious. It's important to remember that when anxiety strikes, your capacity for higher reasoning goes off-line. You can't talk yourself out of how it feels; you can't reason with your brain at that point. Logic isn't going to work, so instead you need to speak the language of the body and give the mind something to focus on.

When you feel anxious, do your best to find a place to sit down away from the noise and movement of other people. Start to shift your breathing so that it is traveling just through your nose. You need to use your breath to signal to your nervous system that all is well. To do this begin to count the beats of your breath. Breathe in for a count of four, and breathe out for a count of four. If your breathing is fast and shallow, do not worry. It will take a little time to for the signals to be received. That's OK. Keep counting your breath and work on bringing it down into the bottom of your lungs so that you feel your belly expand as you inhale and retract as your exhale. You're doing great. Now see if you can breathe in for a count of four but breathe out for a count of six or even eight, pausing for two beats before the next breath in. Notice the belly move as you breathe. In for four. Out for six. Pause for two. Do this for as long as you need to.

As your breathing slows and your chest relaxes, think back through some of the details of one of your favorite stories. Think of how something looked, tasted, or smelled. Stay with those bits of sensory experience. We are moving your attention away from the source of the anxiety and toward that bank of safe places in your own imagination.

The more you do this, the better you will get at it. You will start to accumulate evidence that you are able to quickly and comfortably calm and center yourself. You will start to think of yourself differently—not as a person with anxiety but as a person who knows how to calm down when anxiety happens. Well done. (And know that sometimes more help is needed in treating anxiety. Doctors and therapists and medicine are all useful, so please seek more assistance if you need it.)

· · · · ·

Now you're ready to start reading. The stories in *Nothing Much Happens* are laid out chronologically across the seasons. You might want to start with a story that mirrors the season you are in or maybe the season you are longing for, or you may decide just to start at the beginning—it's up to you!

These stories are all happening in the same universe, in what I call the Village of Nothing Much. The owner of the bookshop might buy a pie from the bakery and hold the door on her way out for the couple that visits the cider mill and so on. As you discover the people and places in the book, you can explore the map on the next page, showing you a bit of the layout of this cozy little city. Come back to it as you read and imagine yourself walking along the streets. This will help you build the world of Nothing Much a bit more solidly into your imagination.

As you read, you'll notice that stories that feature romantic partners don't use gender markers; I write this way so that you can imagine yourself and your own life as unfolding in the stories.

Along the way you'll also find a few extras. There are recipes and meditations and even a couple of crafts, all there to help make this world your own. There is also an index at the end of the book so you can search for a story based on your own favorite cozy criteria.

Now, settle yourself someplace snug and get as comfortable as you can. You're about to head into the world of Nothing Much. It's a friendly, familiar sort of place, with lots to savor and enjoy. Let's all take a deep breath in through the nose, and out through the mouth. Again. Breathe in, and out. Good.

Sweet dreams, my friends.

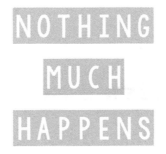

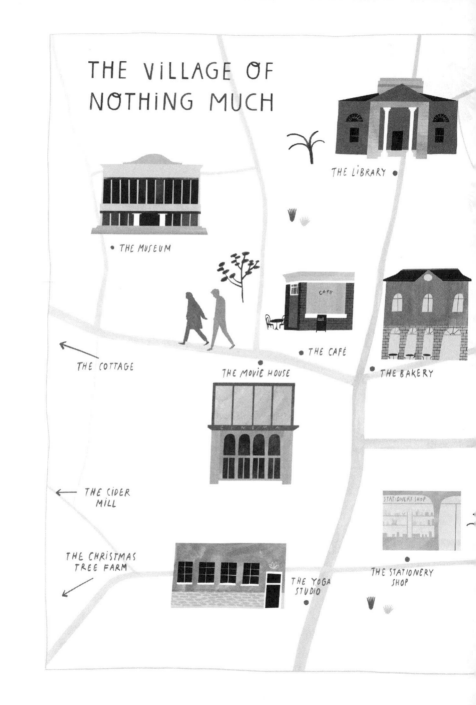

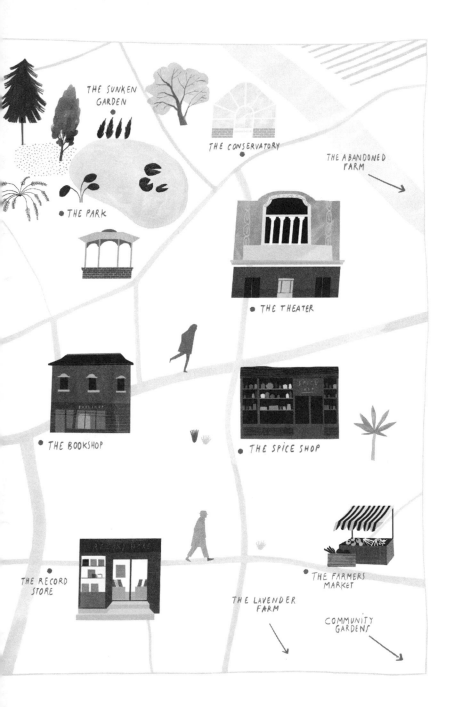

THE SUNKEN GARDEN

THE CONSERVATORY

THE ABANDONED FARM

THE PARK

THE THEATER

THE BOOKSHOP

THE SPICE SHOP

THE RECORD STORE

THE FARMERS MARKET

THE LAVENDER FARM

COMMUNITY GARDENS

Winter Walk

Deep snow had fallen overnight and the morning broke clear and cold.

I lingered at the kitchen table with an extra cup of coffee as I watched the light shift and the sun come up. Sunrise in deep winter, with its bright pinks and streaks of yellow, feels like an affirmation from Mother Nature herself. Yes, the days are short and the landscape coated in shades of white and gray, but the skies are vibrant. There is vibrant life in the thickest days of winter.

With the sun up, I opened all the curtains and let it slant into the rooms of my house. We hadn't seen much sun in a while, and as I began my morning chores, I found myself stopping to look out and taking a few deep breaths.

Someone told me years ago that you get a better night's sleep in a bed that's been made—something about the feeling of tidiness and order helps you to drift off—so I'd made a habit of it, and it had become a kind of morning meditation. I did it the same way each time and took care with the process. I stacked the pillows on the armchair with a little ottoman in front of my bedroom window, where I sometimes sit and read, and I pulled back the duvet and sheet. I smoothed out the sheet underneath and pulled the blankets back up, walking around the bed and refolding and tucking the edges, then shaking out the pillows and plumping them back into place. I took a soft plaid throw that my kitty liked and swirled it into a nest and placed it at the foot of the bed for her. With curtains open and the morning light coming in, the room looked neat and inviting. I had a morning and an afternoon to enjoy but I was already looking forward to going to bed tonight.

With my chores done and the day becoming as warm and bright as it would likely get, I decided to bundle up and take a long walk in the fresh snow. I layered on a sweater and coat, thick socks and boots, a hat and scarf and gloves, and closed the back door behind me. As I began to walk, I looked out at the unbroken drifts of snow, at the peaks of old evergreens and the bare branches of maples stacked with a foot of snow. Winter walks are slow walks; you make your way carefully and a bit ploddingly, but they give you time for lots of thinking and noticing. Past the edge of the yard, I stepped onto a well-worn path and into thickening woods. I had a few acres, and this portion of my land backed up to more woods that were public lands, so I could walk for a long time and not run out of trees and wilderness. I remembered the winter walks I took with my family as a child. There was an empty lot at the end of the street and beyond it fields and clusters of trees, and while the whole thing was probably no bigger than a city block it felt like a secret land, a place where there was no end of exploring to be done. Children have this power, to look at something simple and everyday and imagine the wondrous.

I felt a growing warmth in my belly and chest from the exercise, and I inhaled deep breaths of the fresh air, letting it fill my lungs. The familiar paths looked new in the thick snow and I took a few turns, intentionally leading myself away from my usual route, knowing I could follow my boot prints back if I got turned around. I followed a frozen creek with just a trickle of moving water, and I walked past a thick grove of birch trees, their rippled white bark at home in the white winter, to an open meadow.

I had a sudden feeling that there was something there to see, so I stood still. She stepped out slowly from the trees across the field. A doe, tall and elegant. I guessed she'd seen me long before I was aware of her, but she'd trusted me and let me see her anyway. I was caught by her beauty and stood still and forgot to breathe for a moment. Then I called out, low and calm, "Nice day for a walk," and she wagged her white tail and bent her head to nose through the snow for a bit of winter browse. I supposed she was as glad to see the sun as I had been this morning, and I reminded myself that we all have the earth in common.

I left her to her meal and followed my tracks back through the woods and eventually into my own garden. The long walk had made me hungry and I was already thinking my way through my fridge and pantry and mentally setting the table. I kicked the snow from my boots and stood in the back hall, reversing the process that had started this morning's adventure. I went to my room to change snowy layers for warm fresh ones and found kitty curled into her spot on the bed. She turned her chin up in an impossible angle, wriggled lazily on her spine and let out a soft meow. I curled up around her and told her about the deer I'd seen in the open field. I told her she was probably back in her den by now, nestled down with her friends, and kitty purred. It was good to go out in the woods and walk and remember the fresh air, and then it was good to retrace my steps and tuck back into the warmth and comfort of home. The winter wasn't over yet but the sun was out, and there was much to enjoy while we waited for spring.

Sweet dreams.

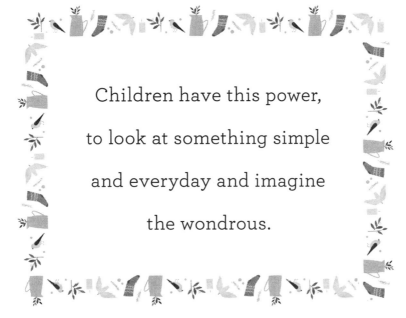

Children have this power,

to look at something simple

and everyday and imagine

the wondrous.

A WALKING MEDITATION

. • . • .

There are lots of ways to meditate. You can practice in a traditional way, seated on a cushion on the floor. Or you can sit in a chair or lie down anywhere that you're comfortable. But some days you might feel like adding movement to your meditation, especially when your mind feels very busy. On those days, try this walking meditation. You can do it inside or out.

Find some clear space, say, 10 to 15 feet. Since this exercise can look peculiar, you might want to pick a spot with some privacy. If you need some assistance with balance, find a space where you can walk with a wall at your side.

Begin standing with your feet situated under your hips, about 8 inches apart. Lift your toes, spread them out and set them back down. Feel your weight shift slightly forward so that your pelvis is balanced over the arches of your feet. If you are barefoot, notice the texture and temperature of the surface you are standing on. If you are wearing shoes, feel the weight of them on the tops of your feet. It might be very subtle. Lift your shoulders up to your ears and take a deep breath in. As you sigh the breath out of your mouth, roll your shoulders down your back and be still. Gently focus your eyes on a spot a few feet in front of you. Before you take your first step, spend a minute here just to feel the sensations in your body. When we spend a lot of time in our heads, we can get numb to what we feel in our bodies. When we meditate with movement we relearn to feel and be present with our own physicality.

Breathe naturally and keep your eyes open but relaxed.

We'll now break up the next step into three parts. You may never have walked as slowly or deliberately as you are about to, but that will allow you to really feel the movement of each step, and feeling is meditating.

Shift your weight into your left foot and raise your right heel from the floor.

Slowly raise your right foot a few inches from the surface you're standing on and feel the weight in your left foot. Walking this slowly requires more balance, so notice the muscles in your ankle and knee responding and supporting you.

Extend your right leg in front of you and touch the right heel to the floor a pace in front of your left foot.

Shift the weight into your right foot. As you do, your left heel will lift. You are back at the beginning of the process.

In this way, continue to slowly work through each step: shifting, lifting, stepping, repeating.

As you walk keep drawing your attention back to what you physically feel in your body. If you find yourself making judgments about the sensations you experience, take a moment to simply label that as "thinking," then go back to feeling. If you reach a point where you need to turn around, do it with the same slow mindfulness you've applied to each step so far.

You may want to set an alarm for ten or fifteen minutes (or as long as you'd like to practice—on a beautiful sunny day I sometimes do this practice for an hour, feeling the grass under my soles and the breeze on my skin). An alarm will prevent you from having to monitor how much time is passing.

When your alarm goes off take one more step and return to the position you started in, feet side by side under your hips. Again, roll your shoulders up to your ears and take a deep breath in. Sigh out through your mouth as you relax your shoulders down onto your back.

Take this mindfulness with you into the rest of your day.

A New Leaf

I'm not one for New Year's resolutions.

After all, why wait for a specific day on the calendar to start something new? All the same, I like reflecting. I like having time to parse a thought or a feeling; to create, sketch, and write; to wander and explore. And the start of a new year is always ripe for that. So when I turn over a new leaf, it's more literal than figurative: I turn the leaf of a new book, or a path on the trail, or a song on a record.

This time around, my fresh start was all to do with a new planner. I still like a physical paper planner, a pretty book in which to write my plans. I enjoy looking at a whole month or week at a time and setting down the dates I'll do the things I mean to do. Last year's was out of pages, and after a year of being carried in my bag and brought out and put away so many times, the hardbound edges were scuffed and the ribbon for finding the day had been pulled out and lost.

So a few days after the busyness of Christmas, I'd found myself on the street in front of one of my favorite shops, looking at the planners in the store window. This little shop has some of the best things: shelves full of blank journals and notebooks just waiting for you to write your great novel in; stationery in a hundred patterns with envelopes to match; sealing wax in a hundred colors and stamps with every letter. They have calendars, some silly with cats doing yoga, and some with the loveliest illustrations of tiny sweet worlds that you can get lost in. And they have planners.

When I stepped in out of the cold, I immediately noticed the smell of the shop, a bit like a library and a bit like a craft room. Actually, it smelled exactly like the library in my elementary school. Have you ever been stopped in your tracks by a smell that took you so powerfully back in time that you had to shake your head to clear it? I remembered the worn blue carpeting of my school, the tall stacks of books, and the excitement of wondering what was in all of them. I remembered pulling an old book off a shelf in a back corner and sliding the card out of the paper pocket inside the front cover to see when it had last been checked out and by whom. I went to a tiny school, which happened to be the same one my father had gone to as a child, and there on the card a few rows from the top, in a child's handwriting, was his name. I guess in a small school it wasn't such a coincidence that we should pick up the same book, but at the time, I remember standing stock-still on that blue carpet, looking around with wide eyes and wondering if the universe had just winked at me. I smiled at the memory and decided that along with my planner I would buy a card to send to Dad.

I started browsing, and before I knew it, I had a little pile of goodies: Dad's card, a calendar to hang in the kitchen, a fresh pack of pencils (I could hardly wait to sharpen them), a packet of origami papers, and my new planner, which had all the features I liked plus a built-in

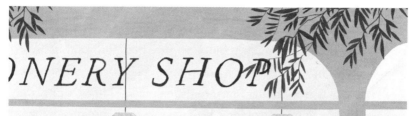
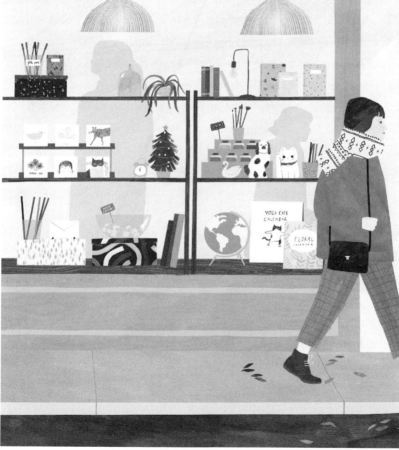

pocket to store some notes and a few pages of stickers in the back. (Was I too old for stickers? I asked myself. Never.) Last in the pile was a new journal. I had so many, and I'd made myself a promise that I wouldn't buy any more till I'd filled up the old ones, so I got only one.

A friendly face at the register rang me up and slipped all my purchases into a bag. As I stepped back out onto the winter street, I thought of the projects I could try out in the New Year, and I walked a few blocks making plans in my head. I noticed a diner with booths lining the window and saw an empty one away from the door. Perfect. I slipped in, pointed to the booth, and a waitress waved me to it. I ordered a cup of coffee and laid my new planner on the Formica table. Then I took out my old planner, along with a new pencil and my sharpener. I'd had a moment just like this a year ago, the changing of the guard. I wrote my name and phone number in the new book, slid my flat palm over the fresh pages, and spun through them, filling in birthdays and appointments and ideas.

The waitress came back to warm up my coffee and she smiled down at my scattered books and pages. "Oh, I love a new planner at New Year's!" she said. I agreed. She went back to her work and I sipped coffee and wrote out Dad's card. I looked through the pages of the wall calendar, marveling at the illustrations. I scanned ahead to next year's Thanksgiving and Christmas, checking where they would land as if I were really planning that far ahead. I guess I was just looking for reasons to daydream about the year to come.

When the street began to get dark, I started packing up my things. The waitress dropped off my bill, and as I was taking out a few dollars to pay it, I thought suddenly about finding Dad's name in that book in the library all those years ago, and how it felt like a little present that had been put in my hands. I took the blank journal, the one I wasn't supposed to buy, slipped a sheet of stickers into the front cover, and left it with the money on the table and went out. I'd written across the bill, "Happy New Year."

Sweet dreams.

In for the Night

I t started as flurries—pretty, lacy flakes that floated down slowly enough for me to see almost each one individually.

I was standing on a street corner, waiting for the light to turn as one large, fragile flake landed in my palm. I saw its symmetrical webs and crystallized branches. I remembered reading that snowflakes formed around a particle of dust. Did that make them like pearls, born from a grain of sand? I liked the idea: a snowflake is a winter pearl, falling from the sky. As I watched the flake, which had been so starkly outlined against my glove, it melted and was gone. These pearls lasted only a moment and needed to be seen before they disappeared.

The light changed and I crossed from corner to corner, catching more flakes in my hands and on my eyelashes. I stepped up to the shop I'd been heading for, and I dusted off my shoulders and cheeks and pulled open the thick front door. I'd found this little shop a few years ago and had immediately fallen in love with their wares, and since then I had become a regular customer. The place sold only spices. Their walls were lined with shelves of tall glass jars, standing shoulder to shoulder, each one filled with something precious and potent, colorful and aromatic. The smell inside was layered, and to take it in properly I stood with my weight balanced across both feet, closed my eyes, and pulled in a deep breath. I could smell the light flowery scents of lavender and herbes de Provence. The next layer down was warmer, with cinnamon bark and cardamom pods. Under that there were complex curry mixtures, the metallic tang of turmeric. At the very bottom of that first deep breath I smelled chilies, hot and sharp and exciting.

I had a list of what I needed, a specific recipe to fill, but I always took some time to look at a few things I'd never seen before and to pick out one new spice to take home with me. I strolled through the aisles and ran my finger over the paper labels on the jars. Some I just liked the sound of, like the grains of paradise, which come from West Africa and are related to ginger and similar to cardamom. Or the fennel pollen, also called the spice of the angels and whose label said could elevate any simple dish into extraordinary cuisine. I opened a jar of amchur powder, which was made from unripe mangoes that had been dried and ground and was used for its tartness. It smelled fruity and tangy but also a little dusty, and I screwed the top back on and kept looking. There were juniper berries that take three years to mature before they can be picked, and bright red smoked paprika, and delicate threads of saffron. There was something called bishop's weed, and nigella seeds, and a tall jar of Kaffir lime leaves. I'd read about these leaves and how they could flavor soups and stir-fries, and I decided this would be my new treasure to take home.

With my new purchase decided, I took out a list from my pocket and started searching for the spices I needed to make my very favorite chai. I'd been trying different chai recipes for a while and had finally landed on a favorite; it was sweet and spicy in a way that warmed me through on a snowy day like today. I had fresh ginger root, cinnamon sticks, and cloves at home, so that was sorted, but I needed cardamom pods, black peppercorns, star anise, and a couple nutmeg seeds. I measured out each ingredient into small paper envelopes, carefully sealing their tops shut as I went, and thought of the collection of tiny former jelly and mustard jars cleaned and drying on my dish rack at home, waiting to house my new spices. My purchases were wrapped and paid for, and I took one more breath of the spicy exotic air and went back out into the snow.

It was picking up now; those light lazy flakes had become a steady falling curtain and the sidewalks and street signs were coated in white. I pulled my scarf up a bit and my hat down a bit and picked my way carefully back to where I'd parked my car. The roads were just beginning to get a little slippery, and I went slowly along the avenues until I was turning into my own driveway. I'd have some shoveling to do later, I supposed. Inside I set my spices on the counter, and as I hung my coat by the door I looked out at the snow falling thickly on the houses around me. I decided I was in for the night. It was such a lovely feeling to watch the snow drape itself over the rooftops while I was safe and warm inside, with no need to go out again.

I thought I might try making a spicy brothy soup with the lime leaves I'd bought. Something with rice noodles and thinly sliced vegetables and a drizzle of sesame oil on top. But first I would transfer all my new spices to their glass jars and make a pot of chai to sip on while I worked. I'm someone who believes that simple chores like cooking and cleaning can be quite enjoyable if you do them right. Light a candle, pour a drink, turn on some music or an old favorite movie, and enjoy the process of taking a task from start to finish in a calm, deliberate way. So I lit my candle and put on a record. I tied my apron around me and started to measure out my spices and dump them into my pot. When the chai was frothy and simmering and the Darjeeling had steeped long enough, I poured out a cup and carried it to the back window, where I could see the light fading, the sun setting behind clouds, and flakes falling onto branches. I stood with my feet planted, like I had in the shop. Tipping my nose down to my cup, I took in a deep breath of the lovely sweet and hot masala of spices before taking a long slow sip.

Sweet dreams.

For the Love of Words

W hen I was a child, I was given a notebook.

It had been almost square and small enough to tuck into my pocket. It had a cover of thick board wrapped in velvet, silky lined pages, and a ribbon, on the end of which dangled a small golden pencil. I'd been shy about writing in it at first; it was so lovely and I was nervous about spoiling the pages by writing the wrong sort of thing. So for a while, I just carried it with me, carefully shifting it from coat pocket to knapsack to bedside table drawer until I finally realized that I was being silly. The same way that trees want to be climbed and my toys want to be played with, my little book wanted to be written in.

I started by writing a few things from my days. I wrote about games I'd played on the playground and the new pair of shoes I'd gotten that I was supposed to wear only on special occasions but which I'd been secretly putting on for solo dance concerts around my bed. I wrote about swimming at summer camp, birthday parties, and what I would be for Halloween. Soon my book was full and I replaced it with a new one. I wrote about sleepovers and science class and my first crush and my first broken heart. In the next book, I wrote about my first after-school job and meeting new friends and the summer concerts we watched stretched out on blankets in open-air arenas.

Each time I filled a book, I'd slide it onto my bookshelf and start another. Through all these years I'd never lost the habit and now had a whole bookshelf just for them, lined up in neat rows starting with that first velvety journal.

I'd gone through phases over the years, sometimes writing less about the day-to-day news of who did what and when and where and writing instead about books I'd read or ideas I'd been pondering. I had a book of recipes I'd tried, noting whom I'd cooked them for and what we had talked about while we ate. I filled one book with all the memories my grandmother had of her own childhood and pasted in photos she had given me, with names and dates written in the margins. I had one full of well-intentioned but poorly done sketches that I'd never shown to anyone and probably never would. That was the lovely thing about all those books on the shelf; they didn't have to add to up to anything. They were just for me, for the pleasure of filling up, and written only for their own sake.

I'd found a word for that and it had inspired my most recent volume. The word was *autotelic*, an adjective meaning a creative endeavor that had a purpose in and of itself. I'd written that word in the first page of my newest journal and decided that I'd fill the whole thing with new and favorite words and what they meant. The project had led me to explore new places and things in order to find words to describe them.

I'd been to a barn on a vineyard and watched them raise a few barrels of wine into a loft for storage, and then I'd written in my book "*Parbuckle* can be a noun when it means a loop of rope used to lower or raise cylindrical objects, but it can also be a verb used to describe the same action. So you can parbuckle with a parbuckle."

I watched a documentary on anatomy and wrote "When I feel the touch of my breath moving over the small divot in my upper lip I will think of the word *philtrum*, which is the proper name for it but also sounds a bit like *filter* and makes me think that it is a place where I can filter in good things and filter out bad."

While tending to the wide bowl of succulents in my front window and thinking about how even plants have a necessary season of respite and dormancy I wrote "*Quiescent* means quiet and not active, and it's good for everyone and everything sometimes."

When a heavy snowfall covered everything in sight and I stood in my boots in a deep drift and listened to the way that all the usual neighborhood noise had been swallowed up, I wrote about *circumambient*, which means to be encompassing and on all sides.

I read a book of poems that used lovely flowery language to describe trivial quotidian things. "*Adoxography*," I wrote, "is pretty writing about simple stuff."

I also found many lovely words in other languages that didn't have an English equivalent but happily added them to my growing list.

I spent a day at the animal shelter, taking dogs for walks and dangling toy mice on strings for a few cats, one of whom had recently had a litter of spotted gray-and-black kittens. I got to hold the kittens and lift their soft bodies up to nuzzle against my throat. Later I wrote about the Tagalog word *gigil*, which means an irresistible desire to squeeze something cute.

I went to a school concert with my sister to watch her daughter play her viola with the orchestra. When the time came for my niece to play her solo and the sound of the bow moving over the strings soared beautifully through the theater, my sister squeezed my hand and smiled through proud tears. Later I found a word for it and added it to my book. "*Naches* is a Yiddish word for secondhand joy. Usually the kind that comes from seeing someone you love succeed."

I found some of these words so useful that it frustrated me a bit that we didn't have a version in our own language, and I started a little campaign among friends and family to adopt a few. There was the Italian phrase of *l'altro ieri*, which literally means "the other yesterday" but in use referred to the day before yesterday, and the Georgian word *zeg*, which means the day after tomorrow. When I was making some salted caramel for the holidays and struck exactly the right balance of flavors, I clapped my hands and declared *lagom*, a Swedish word that means something like not too much and not too little.

My book was nearly full, and soon I'd be slipping it on the shelf with the others. I had one last page, room for one more word. I'd spent the day sick in bed, sleeping and achy, and had only gotten up when I heard a soft knock on the front door. My neighbor, having heard that I was poorly, had made a big pot of soup and carried it in to warm on the stove. With it they brought me a sack of tiny sweet oranges and a box of tea to soothe my throat. They'd stayed only long enough to spoon up a bowl of soup and then left me to my supper and my rest.

I opened my book and thought about a word from the Zulu language, a word that is hard to define in English but encompasses the ideas of shared humanity and compassion, the idea that *I* am because *we* are. I swallowed a spoonful of soup and thought about how reaching out to one another is the most human thing we can do. "*Ubuntu*," I wrote. "You can't be human all by yourself."

Sweet dreams.

A Little Romance

I was out on the streets on a bright winter day. It was cold and the snow still lay thick on the ground in the park and piled around the trunks of trees on the boulevard, but the sun was out and there was a feeling of newness and freshness. We weren't huddling, hunched in our coats and scarves, or racing from shop to shop to dive out of the cold. We were, for the first time in a few months, strolling. Taking our time, turning faces to the sun, and tasting just a scrap of spring in the air. And by we, I mean all of us out on the street today. I was alone, but I wasn't. The sunshine was making us smile at each other as we crossed paths, all of us knowing we were thinking the same thing: "This feels good."

I made my way down the main street, hands deep in my pockets, and turned at the corner toward the park. It wasn't quite lunchtime yet, and I had no place to be. There was a newsstand at the entrance to the park, and I stopped and looked through a few papers and magazines. I found a magazine with pictures of mountaintops in South America and busy city streets in Japan. There were fields of flowers and cold deserts at night. I bought the magazine and a book of crossword puzzles, slid them into my bag, and stepped back onto the park path.

The path wound around a pond, still topped with ice, and walking all the way around it took only a few minutes. I stopped halfway through and sat on a bench in the bright sun. A dozen geese, unbothered by the icy water, paddled in the melted puddles of the pond's surface. I smiled at their putty-gray feet and slick black neck feathers. I remembered that when geese were on the ground you called them collectively a gaggle, but when they were in flight, they were called a skein of geese. I wondered what they called us, and, pulling my coat tighter around me, looked down at the bench and saw a sloppy heart carved into the seat. I ran my finger over the groove in the wood and wondered where *M* and *L* were today and if they still put their letters together inside of hearts. I liked to think so; maybe they were all grown up now and maybe they walked through the park and sat on this bench together and looked down at the heart and remembered, laughingly, the days of young love. If so, I should leave them to it.

I pulled my bag back onto my shoulder and finished my circle of the pond, heading down a side street to a little café I knew. Inside the warm air wrapped around me, making me realize how cold I'd been, and I ordered a bowl of minestrone, full of noodles and vegetables in a rich tomato broth. It warmed me from my center and when it was gone, I ordered a cup of tea and slipped a cookie I'd bought at a bakery that morning from my pocket to dunk in my cup. I thought again of *M* and *L* and love and romance, and as I opened my wallet to pay for my lunch, I took out an old folded photo strip from a secret spot behind my library card. It had been taken years ago at a little booth on a boardwalk. Four frames showing two faces, cheek to cheek, then eyes locked on each other's, then a kiss, then a goofy laugh. I remembered that in Italian, a love affair was sometimes described as a story made with someone, and I thought that I had been lucky. All the stories I'd made had made me a little better, a little wiser, a little more understanding and never less openhearted. I folded the photo along its well-worn crease, tucked it back into its home, and left the little café.

The streets were busy with the lunch hour, and as I wove through window shoppers and slow walkers, I noticed a few kids who must be playing hooky from school. Some were brazen and looking around to see who was noticing them being so grown up, and some had their eyes down just trying not to get caught as they stood in line to buy tickets at the movie theater.

The sky was still bright, and I thought about walking more, doing some shopping or visiting a friend who lived on the next block. But then I thought of that magazine of pictures from around the world and that book of crosswords and the way the afternoon sun slanted across the kitchen table in my apartment and of trading in my boots for slippers, and instead I turned toward my own street.

Passing the bookshop, I noticed the owner trying to push a cart of books through the doorway and stopped to hold it open for her. "Sidewalk sales already?" I asked. "Well, it's sunny," she said, and smiled at me. I helped her slide the cart onto the sidewalk, and we turned a few paperbacks around so the titles were easy to read. She nodded over her shoulder to the apartment mailboxes on the bricks beside the entrance to my place. "Looks like you've got something in your box."

Hmm. Sure enough, the flap was tilted and I could see a corner of something in there. I walked over, fished it out, and held in my hand a small red heart-shaped box. A sneaking smile spread across my face, and I opened the box to see a handful of chocolates tucked in red paper wrappers inside. I might have been blushing, so I just called a quick thanks over my shoulder and slipped through my door.

Sweet dreams.

All the stories I'd made had

made me a little better,

a little wiser, a little more

understanding and never

less openhearted.

Fog and Light

I t was a foggy day, and the streetlights, still lit from the night before, glowed in pockets of patchy yellow on the avenues.

I was walking, rain boots splashing through the puddles of melting snow, on my way to a favorite coffee shop. The gray wet weather had been laying me low, but I had a plan for lifting my spirits, and coffee was just the start of it (though an important part nonetheless). The café was a little funny-shaped space of bricks and old wood wedged into the front corner of a busy building. It served just a few teas and coffees, and on the counter a cake stand held wedges of cake and cookies and muffins tucked under a huge glass dome.

The bell over the door rang as I stepped in, and I got in line behind a little girl wearing a red winter cap and holding her mother's hand. She turned and looked up at me, mouth agape, curious with eyes wide. She was out on a school day and glimpsing the busy world of adults that she rarely saw. I smiled at her and she turned around fast, suddenly shy. I wondered if she'd had to go to the dentist or the doctor, and so she had missed school and now was being taken out for a treat. Her mother ordered her a hot chocolate, not too hot, and a cookie from under the glass dome. The little girl carried her cookie purposefully to a little table in the corner, where she sat down waiting for her drink and pointed out the window at a man walking a dog, calling to her mama that the dog had spots and a red collar like her kitty. Already, I was feeling better.

When it was my turn to order I asked for a simple espresso and slid down the bar to wait for it. I love lingering over a big cup of coffee or tea, but the rich taste of properly made Italian espresso can cut through any gray mood and leave me imagining myself in sunny Campania on a fine spring day. And this little shop did make it properly. It was served up in a tiny white cup and saucer, with barely more than three sips inside. An impossibly small spoon to stir in the sugar rested in the saucer, and beside it was a small glass of fizzy mineral water. The espresso cup had just come out of a warmer, so as I lifted it to breathe in the smell, the ceramic was warm on my lip. First, I just smelled, with eyes closed. Then I took a slow sip and I let it rest on my tongue. It was dark and strong without being bitter or burnt, and I let it sink through my system and restore me. I drank down my mineral water, dropped another dollar in the tip jar, and ducked back out into the fog.

I checked in on how my plan was going: so far so good. I'd had a cup of something delicious, and I'd watched a little girl's face when she saw a dog. I thought of the way her eyes had opened wide, a smile in her voice as she called to her mother, and how she'd swung her legs under the table with excitement. My light was already burning brighter.

The next part of my plan took me through a sodden park with ducks waddling across the paths and around the tiny amphitheater, where I'd sat for summer concerts the year before, to a very special place that seemed like a miracle to find in a busy city. It was a conservatory, a small domed building made of glass, and it reminded me for a moment of the cake stand at the coffee shop. I stood and just looked for a bit, noticing how the fog was clinging to the trees, how thick it seemed, like a shawl I was pulling around the park. Was I pulling it? I shook my head at the thought and pulled open the heavy glass door and let the hot humid air hit my face and neck.

I knew, because I'd counted the last time I was here, that this space was home to more than a hundred varieties of or-chids. I stood still in the entryway, closed my eyes, and breathed in the smell of warm earth and the rich va-nilla scent of the blooms. I hung my coat on a hook by the door and started 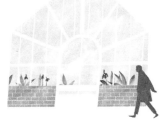 to wind my way through the paths of flowers. The warm humid air felt soft in my lungs and the colors and shapes of the orchids, their varied climbing tendrils and lush petals, pushed all thought from my head. I just looked, and tried not to touch, and enjoyed. I read their names as I moved through and said them slowly, trying to make them stick. *Masdevallia. Brassavola nodosa. Maxillaria. Vanda coerulea. Psychopsis* and *Rhynchostylis.*

I'd had a friend years ago who had lived a long life and was in her final years. She loved orchids, and when I would come to visit, she would show me her collection. She confessed that she'd never really mastered the art of keeping them alive past the loss of their first blooms.

"Oh, well." She shrugged. "I love them so I just buy more and I'll keep at it as long as I'm alive."

And she had. I thought that she would have loved this place and I tried looking at the blooms for her, in her place, as if she could perceive the pleasure of it through me.

Leaving the tiny conservatory, zipping up my coat in the cooler air, I noticed the fog was lifting. There was brightness, a hint of yellow in the sky above me. I slid my hands into my pockets and found in one a peppermint lip balm and in the other a tin box of cinnamon mints. I thought of what I'd learned from my friend's example, the importance of keeping yourself supplied with the small pleasures that made your days a bit sweeter: a tiny cup of espresso, a pair of rain boots to splash through puddles, peppermint lip balm, and days like this, planned to lift a heavy heart.

So many small pleasures to dip into, even while we waited for the first flush of the coming spring.

Sweet dreams.

Getaway

We'd had it in the books since the end of summer, knowing that by the time midwinter came we would need a getaway.

It would be an escape from the bitter cold and gray curtained sky to someplace sunny and hot, someplace with ocean breezes and wild calling birds and hammocks strung from the leaning trunks of palm trees. In the week before we left, I found myself like a child in the last few days of school before summer vacation, coaxing the days forward, crossing them off the calendar at night, and giddily moving through my chores, making light work of packing bags and emptying the fridge.

We moved through the last of the groceries, having a few strange meals of odds and ends: a cup each of the last bit of soup, plates of French toast to use up a loaf of bread, a salad made almost entirely of tiny tomatoes I'd thought for sure we'd have eaten by now, and for dessert, as many bananas as we could swallow. We didn't mind; we laughed over the silly menu and clinked our glasses, each half full of the last bit of wine from the bottle.

When the day came, we were up early, blinking and yawning, quietly pulling on clothes and loading our bags into the car. A long day of travel came next, broken up with winks from one to the other, a secret signal that meant "Hey, we're on vacation," and we'd smile.

Before we knew it, we were touching down and taking that first step out into the hot humid air of a totally new place. It is a wonder of the modern world: wake up in one place, in one season, in one spot on the earth, and then, just a few hours later, be someplace that's quite the opposite, someplace that doesn't resemble one bit the place from which you started.

Soon we were settling in a room with a view of the ocean. It had a vast bed with thick pillows and crisp white linens and a balcony whose door we slid open to fill the room with the sound of rolling waves. We stood leaning out over the ocean, arms around each other's shoulders, and looked up and down the length of the beach, still in our jeans and sweaters from the cold world we'd woken up in. What a feeling to be right at the very beginning of a getaway. The days stretched out in front of us, and we had only to fill them as we went with rest and play, books and dips in the ocean, and walks on the beach. I clapped my hands in excitement. "Last one in the water is a rotten egg," I called out, and we scampered, tossing off our cold-weather gear, rooting through our bags for sunscreen and swimsuits and flip-flops.

Before long we had our routine down. We'd sleep as late as we could manage, order a pot of coffee and plates of fruits and toast and eat them on the balcony with our heels propped up on the railing. Then, we'd dress and go for a long walk up and down the length of the beach, walking hand in hand with bare feet stepping along the very edge of the water, talking or not. Sometimes we'd just stand and look out at the breaking waves, watching birds swoop and dive, fish jump, and families walk and swim. Then we'd find a shady spot, something to sip on, and work our way through paperback after paperback. When the heat built up in our bodies, we'd wade back into the waves to wash it away and splash and play and float till we were hungry or thirsty or ready to go back to basking in the sun. In the afternoon, as the sun was starting to slide toward the horizon, we'd drag our salty, sandy selves back to our room for cool showers on our sun-kissed skin, and then stretch out across the crisp, clean sheets and somehow fall into the third or fourth nap of the day.

Occasionally we'd make a bit of an effort. We'd dress up for a dinner on an open-air patio and enjoy plates of local foods, glasses of wine, or a slow, swaying dance, cheek to cheek, under strings of lights in warm night air. And sometimes we'd gladly order some room service and watch TV through our toes and lie in bed listening to the waves crash on the beach.

As the week waned, I felt myself restored. My skin and hair felt healthy and nourished by the sun and the salt, and I thought I could welcome a few more weeks of cold, snowy days back at home now that I'd restocked my shelves with memories of how it felt to be thoroughly warm and pleasantly worn out by the sun. At home we'd soon see birds returning to nest, rivers swelling with spring melt, and in a month or so, the bare dark earth would break with the first shoots of daffodils and crocuses. Soon after that, the rhubarb would be showing up in the farmers market stalls, and we'd be thumbing through seed catalogues and planning out the garden. I thought I'd like to be back in our own bed again and that it might feel good to have the clothes washed and put tidily away.

How good to have someplace to get away to, so you can step out of the day-to-day for a bit and break all the rules of work. And then, to have someplace just as lovely, though in a very different way, to return to.

Sweet dreams.

A Winter's Day Watched
from the Window

From my front window, I'd been watching what was likely to be the last big snowfall of the winter.

It had drifted in steady blanketing layers over the lawns and rooftops of our neighborhood. I guessed that by now we were all ready for spring but could be talked into one more day of admiring the quiet charm of the falling flakes, one more afternoon pressing snowballs together in our gloved hands and building snowmen, and one more ride on the toboggan down the hill in the park.

I didn't know if I was up for a toboggan ride, but I was up for watching from the cozy warmth of my living room, feet in thick socks and tea kettle starting to whistle from the stove, as a small group of neighborhood kids bundled up to near immobility trundled down the street dragging sleds and saucers on thin ropes behind them. Even in their boots and snow pants they somehow skipped, jogging ahead and calling back to their friends and little sisters to pick up the pace. The sledding hill was waiting.

There'd been a good hill in my neighborhood when I was growing up and I remembered the thrill of bouncing down it, two or three of us crammed together on a sled, holding on to its well-worn reins—and to each other—and shouting out as we picked up speed. We would topple over at the bottom or crash into a heap of snow, and we'd pop up and brush the flakes from our faces and race right back to the top. At some point, either the cold or someone's parent would chase us back inside to warm up. We'd peel off snowy coats and hats and pile them on a radiator to dry out, and, usually before they had, we'd be pulling them back on to head out to the hill again.

I stepped into my kitchen and poured steaming water from the kettle into my cup and dropped in a tea bag, bobbing it slowly up and down and watching the reddish-brown color of the rooibos spread like ink through the water. I went to the cupboard and took down a packet of cookies I'd bought the day before.

I'd been pushing my cart through the aisles of the grocery store, my mind stuck on a loop of busy thoughts from my day, when I'd seen the familiar orange packaging of cookies that I hadn't eaten since I was a child. They were shaped like windmills, a light toasty brown, with flecks of almond spread through the dough. In a flash, I'd forgotten the tangle of thoughts I'd been snagged on and reached out for the pack on the shelf. The lettering was exactly the same as it had been when I was a child, thick and slightly smeared as if it had been printed on an old-fashioned press. Their logo was a smudged windmill and a family name, and as I turned the pack over I saw they were still made in a little town up north. I was suddenly so grateful that these cookies had made their way from up there to down here, onto the shelf of my neighborhood store. I smoothed the wrapper and peered through the cellophane at the biscuits. They weren't perfect shapes, each one a little irregular, some darker or thicker or paler. They'd immediately gone into my cart, and I'd been looking forward to having them with my tea ever since.

I'd eaten these cookies at my grandparents' house. Thinking back, I couldn't remember ever eating them anywhere else. I took out a plate and set a stack of windmills on it and carried them back to the chair by the front window. I settled in, tucking my feet under me and laying a blanket across my lap, and picked up one of the cookies. I brought it to my nose and breathed in its sweet smell. There was a little bit of spice in it—I could smell cloves, nutmeg, cinnamon, and the faint cherry-sweet scent of almonds. I took a bite and the cookie was a bit crumbly and dry, but the taste took me right back to standing in my grandparents' kitchen.

Their house was small, with a tiny front porch, and snuggled into the middle of a stand of towering ancient trees. Because of those trees, it was full of shadows, and the rooms themselves were packed with old pictures and toys that had once been my father's. The kitchen, however, had a big bay window that looked into the backyard. It was bright and full of sun.

My grandmother kept her windmill cookies tucked in the back of a cupboard, hidden behind a canister of flour where my grandfather wouldn't likely stumble across them. She and I would take the packet of cookies to the table, her with her coffee and me with my cup of cocoa, and we'd dunk our cookies, eating them slowly while watching the squirrels race along the power lines. Maybe I'd inherited from her my affinity for quietly looking out windows.

As I looked out on the snowy day, I lifted my cup to her and the memories I had of our time in the kitchen, then washed my cookie down with a slow sip of tea. A few more kids raced to join their friends on the hill, empty mittens dangling from strings at their wrists. I saw the clean way the snow piled up on the bare branches of the sycamore tree in my neighbor's yard and the slanting peachy-orange light that the setting sun was spreading over the sky. Yes, I'd welcome spring when she came, but I was happy to stay snug inside my home for a bit longer and watch the snow fall.

Sweet dreams.

Matinee

hen our children were young, and we'd just moved into this house, we found a friendly group of parents and kids in the neighborhood who were happy to have playdates.

We'd bring all the little ones together in someone's backyard or basement playroom, and they'd run and race, play pretend and dress-up, invent a hundred new games, and build forts from couch cushions and blankets. They'd stop for a snack now and then, gulp down a cup of juice and, handing the cup to the nearest grown-up, get right back to the important business at hand, that of being young and playing.

The children got older, as children do, and soon they were riding bikes up and down the neighborhood streets. They played basketball in the driveway, the steady rhythm of a bouncing ball becoming the soundtrack of most summer afternoons. They'd finish chores or homework and rush out to find their friends by scanning the street for the front yard with three or four bikes tipped over on the lawn. Their games changed, but they hadn't ended. As they grew older and began to head off for their own lives, I realized the lesson I held on to: we must never forget to play, no matter how old we are.

In fact, as an adult, I'd taken to scheduling my own playdates. And though they held some of the same elements those first ones had—there were snacks, sometimes we'd play dress-up, and occasionally pillow forts had been known to happen—they were a lot quieter. Sometimes, I even took them by myself.

Today was one such day. I'd made a plan the night before when I realized a few things all at once. First, I had time off coming to me and that it might as well be today. Second, there was a movie showing in the theater downtown that I desperately wanted to see. And third, across the street from the movie theater was a lovely café whose food I'd been craving for weeks. A movie, all by myself, and a delicious meal—what a treat. I'd gone to bed with a soft smile on my face and woken up full of energy for my day.

I looked at the show times for my movie and saw that there was a matinee right around noon. Perfect. I decided to lounge around for a while in my robe and slippers, then take myself for a long leisurely brunch before the show. There was a novel on my nightstand that needed my attention, so I carried it and a fresh cup of tea over to an armchair by the window, propped my feet up on an ottoman, and began to read. At some point I heard the quiet musical jingle of the bell on my cat's collar and saw the tip of his tail circling through the furniture in the room. In the unhurried way of all cats he eventually meandered over to my chair. He meowed. "Well, come on up then," I said encouragingly. He meowed again. I smoothed the soft fabric of my robe over my legs to show him that he had a spot waiting for him. "Meow." I patted my lap emphatically. How do cats do this? Coming to sit with me was his idea, not mine, but now I was the one nearly begging him to jump up.

He lifted a paw to his mouth and bathed his ears for a few moments to show me he had his own affairs to attend to. I turned back to my book, and after a few moments he sprung up onto my lap. He sprawled out across my legs and I laid one hand in his soft fur. I read. He purred. The rhythm of that purr seemed to echo inside me, and I set my book aside and leaned my head back against the cushion, closing my eyes.

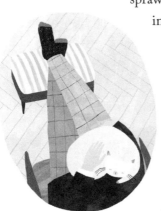

I felt calm and contented. I'd read somewhere that a cat's purr was healing, that it had something to do with the frequency of the vibration; hertz that healed. It released endorphins in both the cat and you. I'm sure there was something to that, but mostly I felt at ease and happy because he did. It was the same feeling I got when I served up a good meal and watched it being enjoyed, or when my children came home from college and I peeked in on them in the morning to watch them sleeping. Seeing those I loved getting the things they needed, well, that was the best medicine I knew.

Thinking of a good meal made me realize that I was hungry. I drank the last sip of tea in my cup and bent forward to scoop up my cat. I set him down in my spot and went to get dressed. A few minutes later, I was stepping out into the cold end-of-the-winter air. We'd had a few days of thaw and freeze while the weather danced back and forth across the edge of the season. There was still snow on the branches and rooftops, but the drifts that had been with us for months were slowly shrinking and the sidewalks were clear instead of icy. I started my car, backed out into the street, and took the long way through the neighborhood out to the main streets.

People were at work. Kids were at school. I was going to brunch. I smiled. Playing hooky is something we all need to do from time to time. I found a spot for the car and strolled for a bit. I stopped at a corner and looked down the avenue at the row of small trees planted in careful grates along the sidewalk. Each one had, hanging from a branch, a heart-shaped ornament made of ice filled with birdseed. I watched for a moment as a small bird stopped to peck at it to free a few seeds. I had a feeling these icy feeders weren't hung up by the city. Someone had made them and strung them with strong twine. They'd come out on a cold day to make sure the birds would be fed and the street would be just a bit kinder.

The café was busy, but not packed, and I found a small round table near a window to sit at. I ordered what sounded good: a stack of pancakes topped with a house-made hazelnut chocolate spread and a glass of pink pulpy grapefruit juice.

When the server set the plate in front of me, I took a moment to savor the way it looked: a stack of golden-brown cakes with a generous dollop of the chocolatey spread and a fan of sliced banana on the side. The sweet-smelling steam rising off the cakes reminded me of fresh donuts. With my mouth watering, I spread a napkin across my lap and started to eat. I ate until I was satisfied, enjoying every bit, and drinking the tart juice last of all.

I looked at my watch, it was nearly time. I paid my bill and hurried across the street to buy a ticket to my show. There were only a few of us there for the matinee and we were spread out in the darkness. I'd picked this movie in particular for today. It was a nostalgic retelling of an old favorite, and it promised to be full of beautiful songs and familiar characters that had been reimagined since I'd taken my own children to see the original many years ago. It seemed likely that I would cry, but while that was nothing to be embarrassed about, I still liked a bit of privacy when I dabbed my eyes and blew my nose. I laughed to myself thinking of my children and what they would make of their mom, planning a good cry for a playdate, but I guessed one day they might feel the same. I checked my pocket for my stash of tissues and then turned my face up to the screen as the lights came down and the overture began.

Sweet dreams.

Spring Rain

The snow was gone and there were moments when the wind blew that I could smell just a little hint of spring creeping out from under the hanging edge of winter.

The days were still short and dark, but with a promise that things were starting to awaken and that a shift was coming.

That morning, a steady rain had been falling, washing out the last stubborn icy patches and soaking into exposed black earth. I'd been inside for too long lately and needed to stretch my legs, and see or hear or think about something new, so I pulled on my yellow rain boots and coat and dug my umbrella out from the back of the closet. It was an old black umbrella, with a carved wooden handle that felt good in my grasp. When I stepped through the front door and opened it up, its hinges and joints creaked a bit, but it expanded to make a huge second sky above my head. I had my own little bubble to walk in and I liked it.

The joy of rain boots is that you can go right ahead and splash as you walk, kicking through puddles and stepping bravely into the muddy spots with as little care as you did when you were a kid. I splashed my way along the alleys and avenues till I found myself deeper into downtown. I didn't have a plan, really; I might stop into a few places but first I just wanted to walk awhile, so I walked all the way down past the park and around the brownstones, watching my feet clapping along the pavement and tilting back my umbrella to let the fresh early-spring air cool my cheeks. Eventually, I circled around the edge of downtown and walked slowly back toward the shops and cafés at its center.

The windows of the coffee shop were steamed up around the edges, the tables inside full of students with books spread out in front of them, and parents with strollers pushed up beside their tables. A man at the stationery shop was hanging a new window display; the winter snowflakes were coming down and big blue raindrops and budding tulips were going up in their place. I passed a bank of windows full of desks with people busily working away. I saw a woman lost in thought, staring out at the falling rain and the umbrellas bobbing past. I had the feeling she wished she were outside in her rain boots with us, and I decided I'd splash through a few puddles on my way home just for her.

There was a record shop on a corner with posters in the windows and just a few people inside looking through the cases, so I folded my umbrella at the door and went in. It was a small, narrow sort of place, with deep wooden bins along the walls and it had a good smell that reminded me of the paperback section of a bookshop. I slipped my umbrella into their stand and drifted for a bit up one wall and down the other, flicking through the albums and sometimes opening one up to look at the art and notes inside. I studied old jazz albums with dark, smoky covers and records pressed this year that were trying to appear old. I browsed through a box of forty-fives, mostly missing their sleeves, and with the names of their original owners written in faded ink. I found an album that my mother had played over and over when I was little, and I was transported for a moment to a summer night when I was seven or eight, standing in the backyard as the sun went down and watching her through the kitchen window as she washed dishes and sang along to the music. I had gaped at her; she was so beautiful.

I carried the record up to the desk and paid for it, and as I slipped my umbrella back out of the stand, I saw a stack of local magazines and papers advertising live music and events. I tucked a few in with my album and headed back to the street. The rain was still falling and I felt refreshed by the cool air as it hit my face. I walked a bit more, my record tucked carefully under my arm, and remembered to splash a little for the office worker dreaming of puddles. I thought about look-ing through a few more shops or stopping to buy a cup of something hot to drink, but I was eager to listen to my record.

Soon I was back at my own front stoop and happy to shed my boots and coat. I shook out my umbrella and left it to drip in the stand by the door. Though the cool air had been wel-come, my warm house now felt like an oasis.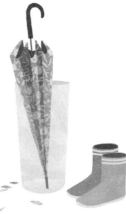

The room was dark in the afternoon, and I turned on the reading lamp by my record player and stooped down to lift the lid. I slid the record out of its sleeve and laid it on the turntable. There was a small cardboard box on the console with a velvet brush inside that I gently swiped over the surface of the vinyl to lift off any dust. The dial turned easily under my hand and the record began to spin. As the needle settled down in the groove and the first sounds of the album began to play, I realized I still knew every word. Singing along, dancing through my living room, I realized I also still knew which song would come next.

Soon albums were fanned out on the floor in front of me, the soundtrack to the rest of my afternoon along with the magazines and papers I'd taken from the record shop, some with dog-eared pages marking a few shows I might like to go to. When the season turns it's important to look forward to what you might enjoy in the coming months, to plan a few adventures, to see or hear or think about something new.

Sweet dreams.

Closing Up Shop

t was just a few minutes till six, and the shop was empty.

I was tidying up the shelves, pushing the books into their neat rows, and switching around the ones that had made their way into the wrong spots. I cleared up the counter, set a stack of bookmarks neatly by the register and locked it. Our little shop had been busy, but now it was finally empty and time to flip the OPEN sign to CLOSED.

The shop was small, on a busy downtown street, in an old building with wide-plank wood floors, tall-coved ceilings, and old wrought iron chandeliers. We had a long counter along one wall that had been there since the place was a hardware store a few generations back, and a wall of windows looking out to the street. There were a few cozy reading nooks with stacks of pillows and illustrations pinned to the walls. You could even bring in a cup of coffee if you promised to be careful, and we had several customers who spent their lunch hours quietly sipping and turning pages and sometimes taking surreptitious bites out of sandwiches or apples from their pockets. We didn't mind. They loved books. That was good enough for us.

One of the nooks was set into the front window of the shop, a sort of booth with a wood-paneled top so that you could hide a bit but still look out and watch people on the street coming and going. Inside the booth were maps of Africa, Europe, and cities in Japan; a map of Middle Earth and of the Hundred Acre Wood; and even a hand-drawn attempt at Fillory. (You know you've picked up a good book if there is a map in the front.) It was generally agreed upon by staff and clientele that this was the best seat in the house, and although it was rarely empty, folks respected its value and didn't hover waiting to claim it.

I turned away from my survey of the shop and back to my chores. First, I locked the back door, an old heavy wooden door that was as old as the building with panels and a few panes of wavy glass. I turned the lock and pulled down the shade. I turned off the lights in the back hall and restrooms, pulled the office door shut, and went to the front door. It was thick and heavy too, but it had a screen door that we used whenever it was warm enough, so a bit of fresh air mixed with the scent of the books. As I closed them up and slid the bolt, I smiled at the bell above. I loved to hear it ring in the morning as my first customers came in, but I also liked closing up at night knowing it wouldn't ring again for a bit.

I stood leaning against the door for a while. This was a nice time of day for people watching, and the spring sunlight was making them blink and smile on their way home from work and school. The shop was quiet. We didn't play music because we thought of ourselves as more of a library than a meeting place with books, so all I heard was the clock ticking and the muffled sounds from the street. Admittedly, I was making this moment last a bit; I was making myself wait. I loved selling books, being surrounded with them and talking about them,

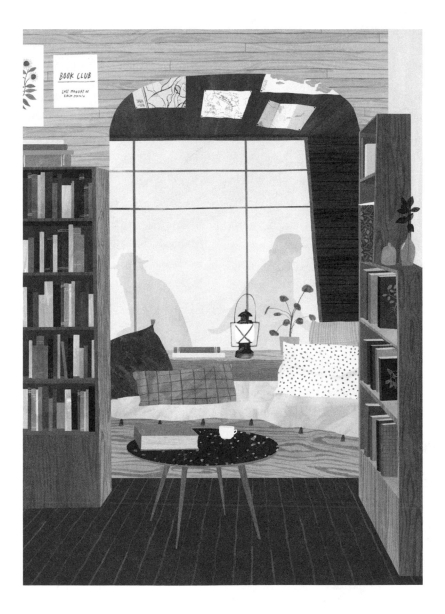

but I also loved being alone and reading them, and at the end of the day that's what I did.

I was enjoying the anticipation as I walked back to the small cluttered office. Inside was an electric kettle, some mugs, and a couple of cookies that a customer had brought me after we'd spent an hour picking out a cookbook together the week before. I flicked the switch on the kettle and pushed the boxes of tea around, finally choosing a box of cinnamon chai. The office had a tiny fridge in the corner and I kept a generous supply of almond milk in there, as it was everybody's favorite for adding to tea. I stirred some sugar into the milky tea, picked up my packet of cookies and my book, and went to the window seat. I was about to begin the second book of a series. I'd loved the first book and had waited more than a year for the volume that was now in my hand. You can only read a great book for the first time once, so I was leaning into the expectancy.

I took my time settling in, making sure to find the right spot for my tea and cookies and the pillows at my back. Once everything felt just right, I pushed off my shoes and stretched my legs out long over the seat, sipping my tea, nibbling a cookie, and looking out the window for a while longer.

Then, I drew a slow deep breath in, sighed it out, and opened my book.

Sweet dreams.

The Asparagus Patch

T he spring air was warm and sweet this morning as I drove through the hilly bare farmlands outside of town.

I was on my way to spend some time with my grandfather, who still planted a full garden each year and kept himself busy around the house fixing broken things and reading books and making pots of vegetable soup. The trees were starting to bud and when you looked across the horizon you could see the light-green haze in the branches that feels like the first true sign that the winter is really over and longer, brighter days are ahead. As I crested a hill, I saw a hot air balloon floating above the line of trees. It was close and unexpected and immediately made me smile in delight. The balloon was bright, with spiraling bands of shining fabric that rippled in the air. I could make out a few riders in its basket, and I thought of what they must be seeing today: the orange-pink morning sky, the neat patchwork squares of the fields, the budding trees and moving cars, all from a new and unusual perspective.

Have you ever had a memory that you aren't sure is real? You wonder if perhaps it was a dream except that it feels lived in, in a way that dreams do not. As I watched that balloon rising in the sky in front of me, I was visited by a memory so strong and clear that it seemed to me it must have been real. I'd been sitting on a cliff on a high hill or mountain and the air around me was full of hot air balloons. Some were close and clear and vibrant and others were tiny spots in the distance. There were a dozen or maybe more, and I just sat and watched them moving through the open air. I remembered thinking that if a rope were hanging from one of the baskets it might brush past me and I could grab it and be pulled away on some adventure.

The more I thought of that moment, though it felt quite real, the more I guessed it must be the memory of a dream or a story I'd heard. I couldn't think of where I could have been that such a thing would have happened, or when, or any specific detail around it. The road curved and I lost sight of the balloon, though I kept thinking of dreams masquerading as memories.

As a child I'd been sure that I'd found a secret cavern in a rocky outcropping by the beach. It was a crack in a wall of stone that I could slip through, and inside I'd found an expansive space full of shimmering rocks and waterfalls and shallow lakes. There were stalactites and stalagmites, some of them meeting in tapered points in the middle, and I'd run my hand over their sides, which were bumpy and smooth at the same time. It smelled like salty sea water and humid summer air, and I was sure somewhere around me there was certain to be a treasure chest waiting to be found. I think I'd kept this memory far in the back of my mind knowing that it just wouldn't stand up to much grown-up scrutiny. After all, the lakes we'd visited when I was growing up weren't rimmed with rocky cliff faces, they'd been sandy or edged with leafy trees, and they were filled with fresh water, not salt.

I supposed I hadn't wanted to admit that it was all a story, so I'd left the memory, dusty and unexamined, in the attic of my mind for years.

I guess it's a mark of growing older that I don't mind so much now knowing that these vibrant and seemingly real scraps of memory are very likely fiction. When I was young they seemed proof of something extraordinary and magical that existed in the world and I fiercely wanted them to be real, but now ordinary things seemed more magical to me than fantasies of flying or discovering long-forgotten treasure.

I thought of my grandfather, turning a piece of burl wood into a bowl in his workshop—sanding and carving and smoothing till it was ready to hold the yellow-green apples that fell from his trees. I thought of the tree that had grown that burl, the knot of twisted wood that had formed around an injury or infection but produced a beautiful swirl in the grain. People were the same at times, producing something beautiful from a time of difficulty. This seemed magical enough for me.

The road under my tires had changed to dirt, and soon I was pulling my car up in front of my grandfather's house. It was a small place but big enough for him and with a yard and garden many times the footprint of the home. I found him gathering small branches and fallen twigs in the grassy space behind his apple trees. After giving him a kiss on his soft wrinkled cheek, I bent and began picking up the kindling as well. He had a shed filled with seasoned wood for his fires in the winter, and we could add all of this to his store. We talked as we worked, and I saw him struggling a bit with the arthritis that was part of his daily life. His joints didn't want to bend and straighten as much as he wanted them to. But he was a very patient man and we just went slower and chatted to pass the time. He plucked up a horse chestnut from the ground and passed it to me saying "Here; if you carry a horse chestnut in your pocket, an elephant will never step on your foot." Who was I to argue with such wise advice?

When we'd gathered all the sticks and stored them away in his shed, we stopped to stand by the bare patch of dirt where he grew his vegetables, and he pointed out where the rows of corn and green beans would go. He was always trying something new in his garden, and he had packets of seeds to show me inside. I'd brought some bagels from the bakery for our midmorning snack, and we turned toward the house to go in. He stopped and pointed to a wide trench of dirt with a few green crowns poking through. It was a new asparagus patch, his old one having finally given out the year before.

"Well done," I told him. "When can you harvest?"

"Oh, in about three years," he said, and gave me a wink. I watched him walk into his house and I slid my hand into my pocket and felt the chestnut he'd given me. *This*, I thought to myself, *isn't a dream. This is what is happening now. Remember it.*

Sweet dreams.

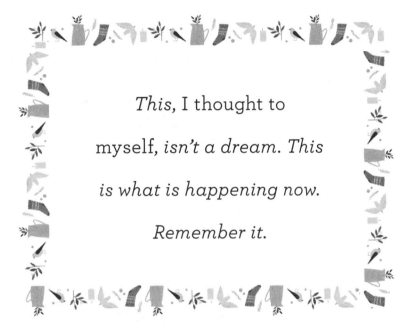

This, I thought to myself, *isn't a dream. This is what is happening now. Remember it.*

First This, Then That

Years ago, a friend offered me a useful piece of advice.

I was rushing, overwhelmed with too much on my plate and starting to gasp and sputter and run out of steam. They reached out and touched my arm, looked into my eyes, and said, "First this, then that." We took a breath together, and I laughed. Their simple suggestion felt like sun breaking through gloom. Of course, I was letting my mind race ahead, and it rightfully felt overwhelmed; instead, I needed to do one thing at a time to find my way from where I was to where I meant to be. Their advice was something I still said to myself when I had a lot of work to get through, but also when I had something to enjoy. It had become a mental touchstone, a method of simply slowing down so that whatever I was doing could be intentional instead of accidental.

I said it to myself this morning, as I pushed aside curtains and lifted blinds in one window after another. The early spring sun was warm and bright and somehow of a completely different quality than the winter sun of just the week before. I couldn't open the windows yet to let the fresh air in—it was still too cold—but I could let the light in and I did. I walked to every window in every room, letting the sun dazzle my eyes, standing in the slanting light and thinking, *First this, then that.*

The house felt different filled with bright daylight, and it made me excited to clear out the remnants of winter with a day of spring cleaning. Not everyone looks forward to days like that, but I do. I like putting things in their place, tidying and organizing and stepping back at the end to see how neatly things can stand. I'd learned a long time ago that when my rooms are disorganized and cluttered, my mind seems to feel the same way. When things are in their place, I feel energized and clearheaded, so I was happy to roll up my sleeves and set my house to rights.

When I'd filled the bird feeders early in the morning, I noticed my coat rack on the way back in. It was covered with scarves and heavy coats and hats with mittens and gloves hanging from pockets and a pile of boots at its foot. I stood in front of it with hands on hips and said, "First this."

I went through the pile, moved coats into the back of the closet, folded away the scarves into a basket, and sorted out the rest. I made peace with my having indeed lost one of my favorite mittens and let go of its lone sister. I felt into pockets and tossed out movie stubs and creased notes. From the very last pocket I pulled out a crisp ten-dollar bill. *Yes!* I laughed aloud at how the feeling of finding money in a forgotten pocket never becomes less joyous, as sweet at ten as it is at thirty or would be (I hoped) at eighty.

Next, I moved through kitchen cupboards, consolidating near-empty boxes of tea and pulling down cookbooks that would be better enjoyed by someone else. We had a neighborhood drop-off for such things, a tiny pantry where you could leave a book you'd finished with, the wok you'd meant to learn to cook with but never had, the sweater that still had a lot of love to give but just didn't fit like it used to. Last week, I'd popped in when I was on a walk and found a little book of poetry by writers I'd never heard of. It was just the right size to slip into the pocket of my spring jacket, and I'd been opening it at bus stops and the line at the coffee shop and reading a few verses.

I'd been filling a handle bag as I worked my way through closets and cupboards and now had a little collection of things ready to find another home. I set it at the back door thinking that, if the sun lasted a bit longer, I could walk it down to the pantry before the day was over.

My work was nearly done; my rooms were fresh and clean and wanting to be lived in. I set the kettle on the stove and lit the flame. While the water heated, I picked through a bunch of flowers in an old ceramic vase on the counter. I'd bought them at the corner grocery a few days before, heavy stems of lilies with some greenery tucked in around them. They were just starting to open and I pinched away the filament and anther. The pollen stained my fingers, and I rinsed them under the tap. I thought of the sleeping bulbs about to wake in my garden, the birds building nests in the still-naked branches, the underground burrows of rabbits growing their families. I thought that spring in Italian was *primavera,* a combination of words meaning "first" and "real." Yes, the year was a few months old by now but the spring was the first real moment of the year.

I took my cup to a chair facing the full bird feeder. There were cardinals and mourning doves and gray jays picking through seeds and hopping in the black dirt. We were all putting our houses in order today. The afternoon light was warm on my skin as I stretched out in the chair. I let my hand reach for a book thinking that I might read a page or two, but the sunlight on my face was irresistibly pushing down my eyelids, and I leaned my head back into the cushion with a slow sigh. My work was done. Now I could rest.

Sweet dreams.

TIPS FOR PUTTING YOUR DUCKS IN A ROW

. . . . .

When you get a day to yourself to attend to the tasks and chores that build up in the background of your life, it can be a real treat to take your time and mindfully move through the work. Here are some tips for enjoying the process.

- Make a list so that you don't have to juggle all the to-dos in your head. Write "Make to-do list" at the top so that once you get to the bottom you can enjoy crossing it off. You're already getting things done!

- If cooking or meal prep is going to be part of your day, pull a couple of cookbooks out and spend some time thinking about what you're interested in making. I recommend making up batches of things like homemade hummus, cooked grains, granola, salad dressing, and soup on days when you have the time. Wash and prep veggies so that salads are quick and easy. And remember that feeling satisfied when you eat is important, so listen to your cravings! If you want a cookie, get to baking.

- Turn on some music or a favorite podcast or audiobook. This is the ideal time for listening to a nice long mystery novel, maybe something thrilling that would keep you up before bed but gets you moving for a day of chores.

- Look for the chores that have gaps of downtime built in and start with those. Laundry for example, has short bursts of active work with big gaps in between while things wash or dry. Making a big pot of rice in a rice steamer or electric pressure cooker might mean you only need to check on it occasionally. Get those tasks rolling and do smaller chores in between. Set an alarm to remind yourself to head back to the laundry room or the stove once a task is complete.

- Work from one room to another as you tidy and organize rather than going back and forth across the house. When you're finished with a particular space, make it feel cozy by lighting a candle, setting out flowers, or turning on low lights so that as you look back you see your progress and how welcoming your home will be when you're done.

Early to Yoga

I was early to yoga, which seemed like a miracle because all day I'd been running behind and racing to catch up.

From the moment I woke up I was tired and a little low, and I'd spent the morning and afternoon fumbling through work and chores. I kept forgetting things, dropping things, and I was getting a bit nasty with myself in my own head. I needed rest and the idea of getting to yoga and laying my mat in that quiet dark space was all that was keeping me going.

And now I was wonderfully early, nearly thirty minutes till class time, but I knew the room would be open and ready. I found a parking spot a block or so from the studio and just sat in the car for a moment. I slid a journal out of my glove box and rooted around till I found a pen. It was a habit of mine to write down whatever was most pressing on my mind before I went in for my yoga practice. This seemed to help me gain a bit of space from my thoughts. Because they existed in the journal, out in the physical world, they didn't have to exist in my head. Sometimes my thoughts behave like a little kid pulling at my sleeve and demanding my attention, and when I put them down on paper, I get a break from that.

I put the journal away, gathered up my mat and keys, and started walking along the downtown street to the studio. I looked in the windows as I went, letting the sights and sounds of the early evening catch my attention. There was an orange dress in the window of a clothing store. There were people eating sandwiches and drinking mugs of coffee in the diner. There were kids playing a game, running along the sidewalks and calling out to each other while their unzipped coats flapped around them in the cool evening air. I could smell wet pavement from the rain we'd had that day, and that fresh black dirt smell that happens only in the spring.

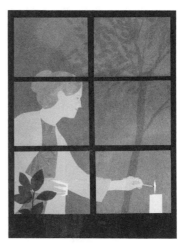

When I saw lights on inside the studio and my teacher at the front desk lighting a candle, I already felt better. I opened the door and slipped in, then quietly took my shoes off and went to the desk to sign in.

"How are you?" my teacher asked.

I took a breath in and blew it out and said, "A bit better now."

She held my gaze a moment. "I see. It's so good that you came tonight. Go put your legs up against the wall."

I nodded, appreciating that I didn't have to explain anything. The yoga room was dark, really dark, with some candles lit and the lights dimmed as low as they could go. The air was warm; it felt easy to breathe and it took the chill from my skin. The room had an orange glow from the lights reflecting on the wood floors that reminded me of sitting in front of a fire. And although I was early, there were already a handful of other students lying or sitting on their mats in the quiet. It reminded me that I wasn't the only one having a bit of a day. No one talks in this room and no one brings their phones in, so it's very quiet, and for the first time today, I felt safe and like I was no longer under the microscope. It was a space where, even though I wasn't alone, I felt like I had privacy and it was good.

I unrolled my mat in the back corner of the room and did as my teacher suggested, sliding up close to the wall, laying my back down on the floor, and swinging my legs up the wall. I immediately sighed. This shape always calms me. I know it has to do with getting my legs up above my heart and the lymphatic fluid blah-blah-blah, but mostly it just feels nice. Minutes passed. I kept my eyes closed. There was quiet piano music playing.

I heard footsteps and then the quiet voice of my teacher near my ear. "Lie all the way onto your mat, I have something that will help." I did as she said and a moment later felt her lay a heavy blanket on top of me. There were little pockets of weights sewn into the fabric and the gentle force of it spread out over me and seemed to press out anxiety and tension. It was like there had been a car alarm going off inside me all day, and I had become so used to the sound that I only noticed when it suddenly stopped.

"What is this?"

"Relief," she said. She smoothed my hair and rested her hands on my shoulders for a moment.

"I might fall asleep," I said quietly.

"Good. I'll wake you up eventually."

I could hear her footsteps retreating and then I just felt the pressure of the blanket, and the warmth and quiet of the room.

Sweet dreams.

RESTORATIVE YOGA POSTURES
FOR A BETTER DAY

. . . . .

Make some room for yourself next to a bit of open wall space. You just need enough room for your legs. You won't need your phone, so leave it behind.

Sit down with your bottom on the floor and with the right side of your body against the wall. Lie back and, as you do, turn your body so that your legs go straight up the wall and your back relaxes on the floor. Your back should now be perpendicular to the wall, with your bottom close to it. You don't need to place your bottom directly against the wall, though sometimes that feels better. Let your hands rest over your belly or let them flop by your side—whatever feels best. Close your eyes and pay gentle attention to your natural breath. Stay here for at least five minutes.

Still at the wall, let your knees bend, and bring the bottoms of your feet together with your knees opening out toward the wall. You might stay here for another five minutes or decide to move on after just one or three. Trust your instincts.

Slide your knees together and slowly turn over onto your favorite side, carefully lowering your body to the ground. You'll find yourself in a fetal position. Stay curled up for a few moments. Let it sink in that you're not in a rush.

Turn away from the wall and stretch out onto your back. Let your toes flop out on either side. Press the back of your head into the floor for a moment, lifting your chest just enough so that you can slide your shoulder blades down your back. Be still and let your body and mind rest for about five minutes. Really rest. No sneaky multitasking behind your eyes. You need rest.

Begin to make some small movements in your hands and feet. Then, take a big yawning stretch from top to bottom. Draw your knees into your chest and give them a good squeeze. Remember that you, like every other person on the planet, deserve compassion and good things.

Turn onto your side, and slowly shift yourself up to a seated position. Move back into your day when you are ready.

Crayons and Grains of Sand

The weather hadn't been able to make up its mind lately. There'd been a string of days with bright sun and warm temperatures, and then a few with driving cold winds and rain that had turned into a dusting of snow. I'd wake in the mornings unsure if I should be layering on thick socks and sweaters or switching them for T-shirts and sandals. Today, I stood for a while and watched the morning light change, waiting to see what color the sky would be when the sun was up. It had started in smeary trails of pink and orange, and I imagined faraway fingers tracing lazy lines through our sky, like a child might do at the edge of a slow-moving creek. Someone had told me once that lines traced on the water disappear the instant they are created and that it might be a useful way to think about my own worries: as something traced in water rather than carved into stone. It had been useful, and looking up at the sky now, I watched the lines blur and fade until they too had dissolved into the dim gray-blue atmosphere. "Still undecided, hmm?" I said to the weather. She didn't answer, at least not right away.

I thought that if Mother Nature wasn't sure what she wanted to do for the day, maybe I didn't need to be either. I wouldn't plan for today;

instead, I'd just follow it moment by moment and see where it took me. My
stomach grumbled and I decided that
the next place it would take me was
my kitchen.

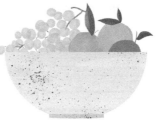

I had a huge ceramic bowl in the center of the kitchen table filled with grape-
fruits, clementines, and satsumas with their papery green leaves still
attached. I'd had a craving lately for fresh tart flavors, so I had stocked
up on all these lovely citrus fruits. I picked up one of the clementines
and held it close to my nose. It smelled sweet and sour, like it would
wake me up a bit. Its peel came off in one piece. I slowly broke off one
section at a time and ate, enjoying the way the tiny packets of juice
burst in my mouth. Next, I picked up a grapefruit. Its skin was an
orangey-yellow with a bloom of pinkish red. This one, I sectioned
carefully with a knife, dropping the half-moon slices into a bowl. I
sprinkled on a bit of dried ginger and cinnamon and got a spoon from
the drawer. I ate slowly; the flavors were so bright and delicious I
didn't want to miss a bit of it. When I set my plate in the sink and
washed the last bit of stickiness from my fingers, I noticed that the
kitchen was scented with the fresh smell of the fruit.

It reminded me of a day in my high school science class when my
teacher sat at her desk and peeled an orange in silence. We all watched,
wondering if the lesson had started or if she was just catching up
on her breakfast. From my seat at the side of the room, I spoke up,
saying how good it smelled. I was rewarded with a smile from my
teacher, who said that day we'd be studying how molecules diffuse

through air, just like the scent of the fruit had traveled across the room to my nose.

Looking into the living room, I noticed that the sun had come out and a shaft of light in the angled shape of the window was drifting across the floor. I thought again of those molecules floating as I watched tiny specks of dust spinning in the sunlight. I went to stand in it for a moment, letting the sun warm my toes, and then my face. The bright sun and the smell of the grapefruit reminded me of a page in my coloring book I'd seen a few days before. I sat at my desk and pulled it toward me. When I was a preschooler I hadn't enjoyed coloring at all. It seemed like something I couldn't sit still long enough to do well, and every page turned into a scribble as I, like a little hummingbird, flew from one place to another. Now, I found it quite relaxing. There was a calming solace to slowly filling the shapes with color and watching the scene on the page before me change. I turned to the page I'd thought of. It was a detailed round shape, with symmetrical designs circling through it: feathers and curlicues and petals. It reminded me a bit of the bowl on my table: the satsumas with their leaves attached, the round clementines and grapefruit.

I opened my big box of crayons and pulled an old coffee mug full of colored pencils closer. I ran my hand over the paper, smoothing it and considering where I wanted to start. Since orange and pink had been the colors of the day so far, I started there. I carefully filled in the designs on the outer edges, alternating between the colors, making something like a bright morning sun. This shape was called a mandala. The book had some that were more intricate and others that were quite plain. Some looked like they were teaching you mathematics with their geometrical designs; others looked like a kaleidoscope of nature, blossoms and buds refracted and repeated in the circle.

I'd had an aunt, a great-aunt actually, who'd worked for many years in a prestigious museum in a big city's downtown area, and she'd told me a story about a group of monks who'd come to create a mandala on the floor of one of its galleries. She described the patient way they'd placed the sand, almost one grain at a time, to create a rich, elaborate design. When they'd nearly completed it, after days on hands and knees working, someone had kicked through it, sending the sand in every direction. My great-aunt turned to look at the monk who'd directed the work. She said it took him a moment, just a moment, and that she could see the calm resolve return almost instantly to his face and then he'd simply said, "It will take us a little bit longer to finish our mandala."

The slant of sunlight had faded, and I heard a faraway rumble of thunder. Mother Nature was changing directions again. The room was darkening, so I switched on a lamp. I reached for new colors: blues and purples and grays and black. I thought of that monk and his way of shifting along with the tides; I thought of times when I'd seen my own best-laid plans kicked apart. I thought of the lines drawn on the water and floating molecules and altering skies. There was a commonality here, something to do with peace and patience around change. I reached for more crayons, deep browns and grassy greens, and thought I'd keep taking my cues from Mother Nature, who hadn't yet made up her mind but was creating all the same.

Sweet dreams.

Three Good Things

All the way at the top of my house, a few steps up and around the corner from the floor below, there's a room just for me.

It's a big open room with windows facing the trees and wood floors with a few worn rugs spread out on them. I have a desk and a bookshelf, a small sofa and a lamp, a little table for doing puzzles or painting, and lots of candles. In the corner, on a soft rug, there is a cushion where I meditate. It's an office, certainly. I get work done there. But it's also a place where I read, listen to music, or just recharge, alone.

Today the house was already quiet, a few windows open on a late spring afternoon. I'd made myself a cup of something warm to drink and climbed the stairs to my room. The trees were budding and I stood at a window and looked out for a while. Sipping my drink, I watched a squirrel sitting in the crook of a branch, her tail flicking every now and then. I set my drink down and checked the few potted plants I had sitting on shelves or windowsills, gave the thirsty ones a drink. Then, I set to lighting the candles. It took a few minutes; it was a sort of ritual. I liked the feeling of marking a moment, and lighting a candle or turning on music or even just taking a big breath all felt like that. I hummed a bit, struck a match, and went from candle to candle until the room had a soft glow and felt cozy and friendly.

I set my cup next to my meditation cushion, then sat down and fidgeted around until I'd figured out where my feet and hips needed to settle for me to be upright and relaxed. I had an old light blanket that I pulled around my shoulders and a bit over my head; I wasn't cold but it made me feel safe and focused. I took a few slow breaths and thought back over the past twenty-four hours. I was looking for three good things. Three sweet moments to relive in my head. I found that when I did this, I reset my brain and seemed to notice more sweetness everywhere I looked for a day or so afterward.

In the quiet of my mind, a memory rose up.

In bed the night before, my sweetheart had rolled over in between dreams and bumped a hand along my arm. Without waking, my love squeezed my wrist and held on. I felt contentment bloom through my body and listened as slow breathing became a quiet snore. I smiled to myself in the darkness until I fell back to sleep. I smiled to myself now, wrapped in my blanket, remembering how good it felt to be touched by the person you love.

I breathed and sat still, looking for another good moment.

That morning, stepping out into the fresh spring air with my dogs, I stopped to pick a lily of the valley from around the roots of the sycamore tree in the yard. The stem was so fine and the tiny bell-shaped blossoms so delicate that I just stood and marveled at it. Spring was filling in the gaps that winter had left in the yard and the air smelled so clean that breathing deep felt like medicine. My dogs sniffed around and chased each other through the grass, and I felt simple joy. Now, on my cushion, I remembered that feeling and traced it back and forth in my mind so that those connections in my brain became lasting.

One more time I dipped into my memory for something sweet.

I thought of a visit I'd made to a friend at lunchtime. She had a new baby, just a few weeks old, and I'd brought by a bag of groceries and offered to hold her little girl while she napped and showered. My friend laid her child in my arms and sneaked out of the room to take care of herself for a bit. The baby was so new that sleep came easy to her and she quickly dozed off. I leaned back into the sofa and rested her head under my chin. The weight of her little body on my chest had felt so good that it was like a drug in my system. I was suddenly calm and content. I tipped my nose down and breathed in her smell.

Sitting in my little room, feeling the afternoon light on my face, I remembered. The weight of the baby, the delicate stem of the lily of the valley, the touch of my love. I held it all in my mind and just sat with it. It filled in places inside me where things had been knocked out or lost. I felt whole and happy and quiet.

Sweet dreams.

THREE GOOD THINGS TO START YOUR DAY

· · · · ·

When you wake up in the morning, lie still in bed. Don't reach for anything; just be. Slowly rewind through the previous twenty-four hours and look for three good things that happened to you or that you witnessed. They can be very small things or very big things. Maybe there was a moment when something could have gone wrong and it didn't. Put it on the list. Maybe someone was kind or patient. Put it on the list. Maybe you took some small step forward in your work, or you found something you'd thought you lost, or you saw a dog and smiled. Put it on the list.

Retrace the feeling of those moments back and forth in your mind. Think of your mind like an Etch A Sketch. Remember using an Etch A Sketch to draw shapes and write words? And how you could trace back and forth a few times to make the lines darker? Do that with the three good things.

Now think of what would happen when you'd leave the Etch A Sketch somewhere, on a shelf or in your toy box, and come back to it later—how, even after you gave it a good shake, there would be a bit of a shadow from those deeply etched lines. Your heart and mind are like that. If you take time to sit with the good things, they won't leave you so easily. Let's make the remembrance of good so deep and rich that even when life gives us a good shake we can still make out what is sweet and hopeful.

In the Bakery

I stood inside the front window of the shop and looked up and down the street for a few moments.

Morning light was cutting through the lines of the buildings and a few of the storefront windows were lit up. The neon sign in the diner on the corner flickered and glowed steadily on.

I knew our customers would start to arrive in a few minutes for their orders of bagels, pastries, and loaves of fresh sliced bread. I dusted off my floury fingers on my apron and flipped our sign from CLOSED to OPEN, before unlocking the heavy oak door and stepping back behind the counter. Our cases were full of just-baked muffins, rolls, and loaves. Our coffee was brewed and I had a hot cup tucked behind the register. We were ready.

Saturday mornings were my favorite at the bakery. During the week, customers rushed in and out, eager to get their breakfast and coffee and get to work. But on the weekends, all of us, bakers and customers alike, were more relaxed. People lingered over coffee, turned the pages of newspapers slowly, and took time to really enjoy the jelly donuts and wedges of coffee cake that we loved to make each day.

The bell over the door rang and I looked up to see the familiar face of a waitress from the diner, her spring coat pulled over her apron, hands ready to receive the tray of goods we had wrapped up and ready.

"In a hurry?" I asked her.

"No, it's Saturday," she said with a wave of her hand. "We've only got a couple regulars who pour their own coffee anyway."

We smiled.

"Well, try this then." I passed her over a slice of still-warm biscotti in a waxed-paper wrap. "I'm trying new recipes and I need an opinion I can trust."

She took it gratefully, and I poured her a quick cup of coffee to go with it. "It's orange and pistachio, and you might want to dunk it," I said, sliding the cup across the counter.

"I don't trust people who don't dunk," she observed.

"This is why I'm asking your opinion," I said, tapping my finger to my nose.

She held the slice up close to her nose and breathed in the cookie's smell. She looked at it all over, and I saw her taking in the ratio of pistachio pieces to ribbons of orange zest. Sometimes when I hand someone a sample and ask them for feedback, they gobble it down in two bites, say "It's great," and move on, which is nice to hear but is not very helpful. This woman knew what she was about. She had a bite without dunking first, chewed slowly, then thoughtfully dipped it in her coffee and took a second bite. She looked up at me, ran her tongue over her teeth, nodding slowly.

"I think the orange should be a bit stronger, but the bake is right on. It's crispy and a pleasure to dunk, but if you want to eat it as is, it's not going to break your teeth like some biscotti will. I'd say it's a winner."

Pleased down to my clogs, as all bakers are when something they make is properly appreciated, I slid the coffee thermos back onto its warmer and went to fetch the order she'd come in for. I handed it over to her, she thanked me for the treat, and we said, "See you tomorrow" as she headed back to her customers.

For the next few hours, there was a steady stream of patrons. Some were regulars whose orders we knew by heart, and some were new faces who stood staring at the cases, biting their lips and asking for recommendations. We brewed pots and pots of coffee, packed dozens of donuts into paper boxes tied with string, handed over plate after plate of muffins and scones and toasted bagels. We handed out soft salty pretzels wrapped in waxed paper. Boxes of dinner rolls and focaccia slid across the counter into eager hands. We sliced loaves and wrapped them up for afternoon sandwiches. Pies were deliberated over and finally selected and names were piled onto birthday cakes. We wiped crumbs from the counter and tables and started to deliver the sad news that this or that had sold out for the day.

As the day moved on and the bell rang less and less, I pulled out a few of my favorite cookbooks from the shelf in the office and poured a fresh cup of coffee. I set myself up at the counter where the sun was shining and flipped through the book that was older than I was, with pages stained and creased and filled with handwritten notes. It was a gift from the baker who'd first opened this shop; I'd bought the shop when he retired. He was a kind man with a quiet voice and flour in his eyebrows. I remembered coming in for my daily bread and, one day,

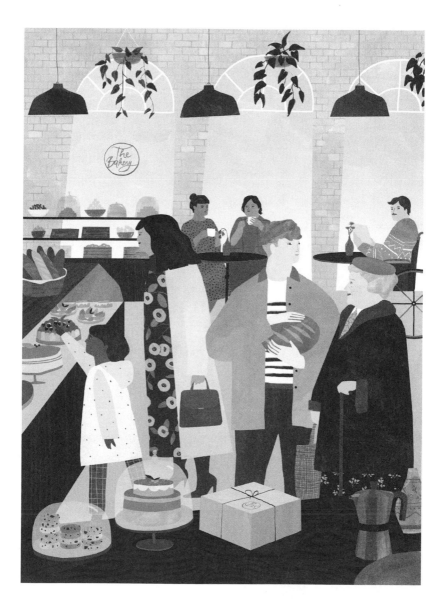

taking a bite of something and saying to him that I could always tell his bakes from any others, that he seemed to have a sort of signature flavor. He'd smiled, leaned his elbows on the counter, and, turning his head side to side to make sure his secret wouldn't be heard by anyone else, he whispered, "graham flour." We'd been friends from that day, and I came to work for him soon after.

Looking through his book of recipes made my stomach grumble, and I stepped behind the counter and took a baguette from the shelf. I sliced off a good long bit and slit it open. I had a bottle of olive oil, green and fruity, the kind that catches you in the back of the throat, and I drizzled it over the bread. In the fridge I found a stash of artichoke hearts and a jar of capers, and in the pantry, a container of soft sun-dried tomatoes. I layered them all over the oiled bread, cracked black pepper on top and took my plate back to the sunny spot at the counter.

My bread was delicious, and I proudly enjoyed every bite as I flipped through more biscotti recipes. I took the pen from my pocket and added a note, "More orange flavor . . . maybe add marmalade?" My next plan was for hazelnut and chocolate biscotti, and something for spring. Strawberry and rhubarb? I carried my cup back to the window where I'd stood that morning before flipping the sign. I looked up and down the street. Saturdays were my favorite.

Sweet dreams.

Spring, at the Allotment

When I'd first seen the flyer, snow was still on the ground.
I'd been coming out of my neighborhood market, a bag of groceries in my arms, when I skimmed the bulletin board. "Community Garden. Plots available!" The flyer was decorated with someone's hand-drawn flowers and baskets of vegetables. I stood for a bit—booted, mittened, zipped into my heavy coat, and wrapped in scarves and a hat—and dreamed about green things and blue skies. I'd reached out with my clumsy mitten and pulled off a scrap with a phone number from the flyer and fumbled it into my pocket.

A few days later, when a friend was sitting at my kitchen table for a cup of coffee, I'd pulled it out and we'd made a plan. Each of us had a few hand-me-down garden tools and just a little bit of experience, but we also had a deep yen for becoming successful gardeners, and we figured

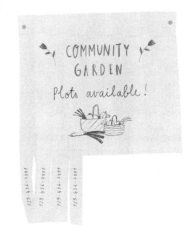

our zeal would fill in the gaps of our knowledge. We'd divvied up the work; she'd go to the library and get us a few books on what was best to grow in our first year, and I'd have a long talk with my green-thumbed grandfather and borrow his almanac and seed catalogs. We'd both root around for gloves and rakes, spades and shears and loppers.

Soon we had a stack of books, with torn-out magazine articles folded into the pages, charts of what was going where and when, a dusty basket of the tools we'd need to make it happen, mud boots, and packets of seeds. We planned to meet at the allotment in the midmorning on Saturday to begin our garden.

The day was bright and warming. Stepping out of the car, I could smell the clean scent of freshly tilled earth. We found our plot, sketched out in the soil with stakes and string, shook hands with the neighbors, tucked our hair into bandanas, and got to work.

The soil was tilled and soft but still needed to be evened out, and we broke up clumps of dirt with hands and hoes. We consulted our charts and walked off the sections. Here we'd plant the herbs: basil and oregano, lavender and rosemary, sage and thyme. Here we'd plant runner beans and green beans, here rows of lettuce, and here tomato plants. In the back, we'd have a line of sweet corn, a section of zucchini, a few broccoli plants, cabbage, cucumbers, and a small section of potatoes. We weren't sure about the potatoes. They seemed tricky, but we'd done our reading and had a container of cut seed potatoes ready to go in. Growing anything, I supposed, was a gamble, an act of faith that rain would come, sun would shine, and the natural processes buried in the cells of our seeds and seedlings would activate and pullulate. It seemed worth the gamble, meriting the faith to try, so we dug trenches, spaced our seeds and plants and carefully patted the earth down around them.

By the time the sun was high above us, we'd shed our jackets and our faces were smudged with dirt. I stood to stretch my back and saw my friend, her hands on her hips looking out at the work we'd done.

"Ready for a break?" I called out.

"Yes, please," she said, stepping carefully through the rows to wash her hands at the spigot.

I'd packed us a basket for lunch and we carried it over to a picnic table and opened it up. I had a thermos of Earl Grey tea, still hot and a little sweet. I'd made a mess of sandwiches, thick slices of sourdough spread with spicy mustard and a mash of garbanzos, soft avocado, diced cucumbers and pickles, tahini, a bit of dill and lemon and plenty of salt and pepper. I'd layered it on the bread with sprouts and tomato slices and wrapped them in tea towels. I also had a few apples for us and a whole batch of my date bars topped with a cardamom crumble tucked in waxed paper in an old cookie tin.

It was more than we could eat, but I'd planned to use the extra to make some friends. In fact, a few minutes after we'd spread out lunch, the family from the next plot over sat down to share our table. They unpacked their basket, and we chatted about our seeds as we ate. They had two little boys who ran around in the sun. Every so often, they would come back to the table to take a bite out of a sandwich or a piece of fruit and then chase each other back to play. The family had been planting in the garden for years and promised to offer advice as the season progressed.

They poured us some of their lemonade, happily took some date bars, and then we all got back to work. By the time we were done and gathering our tools, our little plot was a tidy patch of neat rows, careful mounds protecting seeds that would sprout soon, and evenly spaced plants that would need cages and stakes and strings to hold them up by the end of the summer. We stood and proudly admired what we'd done.

"We'll have vegetables coming out of our ears in a few months," my friend said.

"I guess we'd better learn how to can," I said with a laugh. "The next great adventure."

Sweet dreams.

Mashed Chickpea Sandwich

· · · · ·

MAKES 4 SANDWICHES

These tasty sandwiches are perfect for a picnic. The filling gets even better after some time spent in the fridge, so if you have a chance, make it up the night before. If you're like me and forget to do things ahead of time, throw this together whenever you need a good lunch—it will still be delicious! Feel free to adjust this recipe by adding more dill or less lemon, as desired. And nobody has the right to tell you how much avocado to put into anything. If you want more, add to your heart's content, but remember that it will make your mix a bit mushier and less crunchy.

CHICKPEA FILLING

1 can (15.5 ounces) chickpeas, drained and rinsed

1/2 cup finely chopped dill pickles

1/2 cup finely chopped cucumber

1 tablespoon chopped fresh dill, or 1 teaspoon
   dried dill

1/2 avocado, pitted, peeled, and sliced

2 tablespoons fresh lemon juice

1 tablespoon tahini

Salt and pepper, to taste

FOR SERVING

8 slices sourdough bread or bread of choice

4 tablespoons spicy mustard

4 handfuls fresh sprouts, such as alfalfa or broccoli

To make the chickpea filling, place the chickpeas in a shallow dish. Using a fork, mash the chickpeas. Make sure you don't pulverize them, just break them up and leave a few whole so there is some texture to the mix. Add the pickles, cucumber, and dill, and stir until evenly distributed through the chickpea mixture.

In a small bowl, use a fork to mash the avocado until smooth. Add the lemon juice and tahini to the mashed avocado, and stir to combine. Stir the avocado mixture into the chickpea mixture. Season with salt and pepper, to taste. Store the chickpea filling in an airtight container in the fridge for up to four days.

To assemble the sandwiches for serving, toast the bread. Arrange the slices on a large cutting board or clean surface.

Spread four of the slices with the mustard. Pile about 1/2 cup of the chickpea mixture on each of those slices. Top each with a handful of sprouts. Place the remaining slices of toasted bread on top.

Wrap each sandwich in a clean tea towel. You can make these up a few hours before eating, but they are best eaten soon after they're made. When it's time for your picnic, pack them in a basket and tote them with you to your favorite spot. You're gonna make some friends with these sandwiches.

Opening the Cottage

I t is perhaps a distinction that not everyone will agree with, but as far as I am concerned, cabins are in the woods, and cottages are by the water.

A cabin might live in a shady glade, tall pines or ancient oaks standing close by with branches curling overhead. It might have dark paneled walls and a wood burning stove for warming feet in thick socks. It is the best place to be on a foggy autumn morning or at the first snow of the year, with a cup in hand and eyes on the slowly blanketing landscape.

A cottage sits on the edge of a river or by a broad lake. Its walls are painted a faded shade of yellow or white; it has weeping willows for neighbors, their buds the first to go green in the early spring. It is the best place to be on the cusp of warm months, with a glass of iced tea in the afternoon and eyes always on the moving water.

And so, we were on our way, to open the cottage. The car was packed with a few days' worth of clothes good for cleaning and walking, paper grocery sacks of provisions, a couple of dogs, and our giddy selves. The drive was familiar, routes we'd been taking for years, and we passed the shop we sometimes stop at for iced drinks and sweet corn in the late

summer, the little town
with one stoplight and
the old depot over-
grown with ivy and
wisteria. We turned
on the state road, cir-
cled past the house with

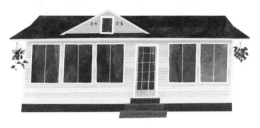

shrubs cut to look like animals and train cars, and kept going just a bit longer, till the air started to smell different. Finally, we leaned forward in our seats, squinting a bit, to catch sight of the front porch and familiar trees of the cottage.

It was an old place built at the beginning of the last century, with white clapboard siding and a front full of windows. As we pulled up, the dogs danced in our laps. They knew where we were and were as excited as us too. When we opened the doors, they jumped down and started a determined sniffing investigation of every blade of grass. They were checking the guest book, as it were, seeing who exactly had passed through since we'd closed up in the fall. We let them sniff and did our own bit of inventory, checking for loose screens in the windows. We noticed a few branches that had fallen on the roof during a storm and the buds of lilacs on the bush.

As we stepped up onto the front porch, the dogs rushed to follow us in, their whole bodies wagging now, noses pressed up against the crack under the door. I found the key on my ring, the one with a tiny red heart dabbed on in nail polish, and wiggled it into the lock. When I pushed the door open, the dogs shot through the place, running from room to room, and we started to pull back curtains, roll up blinds, and open windows. Under the closed-up musty smell, I could already detect the scent that was so deeply tied into this place. It was like old wood warmed in the sun, like old books and the cases they've lived in for years, and with it was the smell of fresh water and hundreds of breakfasts cooked late on Saturday mornings. It was simply the best smell in the world.

Once the car was unpacked and the dogs had worn themselves out with sniffing and found spots in the sun on the front porch, we rolled up our sleeves and started to work our way through the little house. We put fresh sheets on the bed and swept the floors. We stocked the kitchen cupboards and filled the fridge. We put clean towels in the bathroom and wiped the dust from every surface. We frowned at the fuse box and water heater and flipped switches until we'd figured it out.

"We should write down how we did that so we have it for next year," I said.

"Mm-hmm."

We both knew we wouldn't. It was part of the tradition.

We strung up the clothesline in the backyard, glad to think that soon it would hold exclusively beach towels and swimsuits. We waved at neighbors, called out hellos and how-are-yous. There was more to do, but we'd done all we wanted to for the day, so we stood shoulder to shoulder in the kitchen and fixed some sandwiches, then carried them out to the water. We walked to the edge of the dock and sat down with our legs dangling over, toes a few inches away from the still-chilly flowing river. We'd been saving this moment and we both knew it.

Is it this way for everyone? Does the water call you like home? Do you get antsy and edgy when you're away from it for too long? Do you feel restored when you're back on its shores? Maybe it's because I grew up here—because I've slept on the front porch swing a hundred times as a kid and jumped off this dock in every year of my life since I could walk. Or does water pull everyone the same? If I'd grown up in a dessert, walked dunes of dry sand, and celebrated the days of my life in the rare shade of palms, would I feel called by the arid heat?

Beside me, an arm was raised and a finger was pointed down the length of the river at a long dash of steel in the distance.

"Ship!"

"Ship!" I said back.

We'd see a hundred before the summer was over, but it never stopped being exciting. Some we knew well, having seen them for years, their entries well thumbed in the ship's book; we knew how long they were, what they carried, and could see just by looking at them if they were full or empty of cargo. This one, however, looked brand new, fresh paint and sleek lines. I looked forward to hearing the ship horns in the night, to seeing their lighted bows and sterns slipping through the black water. There was no sleep like cottage sleep, and no waking like cottage mornings.

We heard the paws of the dogs behind us as they crept down the dock to sit beside us; a furry head came to rest on my thigh and I slipped my hand over the dog's shaggy ear and stroked the spot between her eyes. We were all quiet together, just looking out at the slow-moving ship, the wake building at its bow and the waterbirds overhead. I was sure that cabins held their own joys, but this was a cottage, and it was the best place to be for the summer.

Sweet dreams.

MEDITATION BY THE WATER

· · · · ·

Start just by standing near the water. Place your feet about hips' width apart and feel your weight shift a bit forward over your arches. Relax your hands to your sides and close your eyes. Take a slow breath in through your nose and then sigh it out of your mouth.

Notice what you can hear in the space around you. Maybe the water is moving and making some sound; maybe there are birds or insects or other people. Without forming any opinion on what you are hearing, just listen to the sounds themselves. Be curious about them: notice volume, rhythm, and even which ear a sound is landing in.

Slowly open your eyes and focus on a single aspect of the landscape. Maybe there is a tree or cloud or boat in the middle distance. Again, without forming any opinions about what you are looking at, just notice the shapes and colors and textures. Then, let your eyes roam over the water, noticing how it ripples and flows.

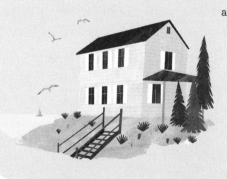

Spend a few more minutes feeling the weight of your body balancing over your feet, hearing the sounds around you, and looking at the sights. Meditation is simply paying attention in a calm way. You've done that. Take one more deep breath in through your nose and out through your mouth. Good.

The Lilac Thief

There are only a few days of spring when you can step out of the door and smell lilacs on every passing breeze.

They're bright and sweet and there's nothing to do but plant your feet and take slow deep breaths to try to store their scent deep inside for another year.

The lilacs.

I remember, as a child, pressing my face into their soft blooms, dew coming away on my cheeks, and wondering how something could smell and look like that and grow so abundantly and be . . . allowed. It seemed too good, too perfectly aligned with what was pleasing to just occur naturally. But I guess there is a catch with lilacs. They bloom only once a year and they don't last long. In fact, they're best enjoyed on the tree; when you cut them and bring them inside, they soon wilt and dry up and their sweet smell fades.

Still, I couldn't help myself. I would try to be surrounded by them for as long as possible each spring and that meant taking matters into my own hands and possibly some very gentle trespassing. You see, I am a lilac thief. I don't strike at random; my crimes aren't ham-fisted or even much noticed. I'm a subtle thief; I plan when and where and make my getaway before anyone is the wiser. When I walk my neighborhood, I might casually reach up for a stray blossom creeping through the slats of a fence and just as casually tuck it into the flag of a mailbox for someone to find later, but I know better than to pull a real heist so close to home.

For that I packed a kit into my car (wicker basket, garden gloves, twine, and a small set of pruning shears), dressed inconspicuously, and drove into the countryside. There was an old farmhouse, long since abandoned, on a dirt road that I knew well. I'd cased the joint years ago and found the house reliably empty and the yard reliably full of lilac trees. I parked my car on the edge of the road to give myself a bit of plausible deniability; after all, perhaps I'd just had a bit of car trouble and was letting an overheated engine cool down and had stopped to smell the roses as it were. I chuckled to myself as I took my kit from the back seat, master criminal that I was, and made my way down the long and dusty drive that led to the old house.

I stood with the sun on my face for a few moments and let my imagination spin a story about who might have lived here. I thought of kids running through the vegetable patch, a pack of family dogs racing with them, sparklers on the Fourth of July, a kitchen with rows of freshly canned pickles laid out on cotton towels, a tree planted to mark a special day a hundred years ago that grew to the one I looked at now. The house had a large wraparound porch, and though the stairs had a few missing boards and the paint was chipped and faded, I could tell it had been a beloved place in its time.

I followed my nose to the large row of lilacs and put on my gloves and opened my shears. The blossoms were so full and heavy that their stems struggled to stay upright. I set my basket down and started to relieve them of their burden. I took time to notice each small bloom, drink deep the smell, and patiently wait for bees to shift from one flower to another. I filled my basket till it nearly overflowed, and still the trees seemed as full as they had been when I started. I kicked my way back down the drive and with a surreptitious look up and down the road, I smuggled my goods back into the car and made my getaway.

All that stealing had made me thirsty and I was craving a cold brew coffee from a little café near my house. I decided to bring my basket with me and found a seat at a tiny table outside. I ordered my iced coffee with a bit of coconut milk and sat my basket on the seat beside me. I picked through the stems, making small bouquets and tying them up with twine. Some were for me, and some I'd leave on the doorsteps of friends.

"Did you steal those lilacs?" asked a voice from behind me.

I turned to see an older man, with gray hair and bright eyes looking at me over his cup of coffee.

"What lilacs?" I asked innocently.

He winked at me and touched his finger to the side of his nose.

"Takes one to know one."

I laughed out loud and passed him over a bundle of flowers. He pressed them to his face and took a deep breath in and let it out in a contented sigh.

We chatted for a few minutes about some of our favorite spots. He told me about a place by the highway, and I told him about the tree behind the library. He lifted the bouquet to thank me, and I carried my basket out to divvy up the rest of my plunder among friends and strangers on my way back home.

Sweet dreams.

Coffee on the Stoop, or
How to Have a Better Day

T he day was dawning.

I looked out at the bright blue sky behind a layer of alto-cumulus clouds, the kind that look like the rippling surface of a lake on a breezy day. My coffee sat beside me, steaming in the air on the front stoop, and the roasty-rich smell mixed with the green scent of grass and growing gardens. We'd had warmer days in the last few weeks, but we hadn't had a warm morning until today, and somehow I had woken up knowing it. Maybe I could smell it through the tiny crack in the window or maybe I could hear the birds singing differently in the warm air, but before I opened my eyes, I knew the morning would be sweet and bright. And it was. I sat with no plans, sipping slowly and watching the sky change. Across the street I watched my neighbor's kitty, a Siamese with fawn fur and deep brown streaks around her eyes and ears, pace across the top of the sofa in her front window. Eventually she sat and I watched her watch the birds moving through the branches of the old trees on our street.

I was on my second cup when I finally saw it. A smudged scrap of paper tucked under the corner of an empty flowerpot on the top step of the porch. I lifted an eyebrow and just puzzled at it for a moment. Had I left something there? Maybe I'd dropped a piece of mail or a shopping list had fallen out of my pocket? I shifted the pot and smiled down at an inked note. "Flowers for your porch," it said. Under the note I found three packs of seeds, all flowers, different types and different colors. I laughed a bit and, picking them up, looked up and down the street as though the gift giver might still be there watching me.

It reminded me suddenly of an old friend of mine who was an expert stealth giver. She had once hidden some small trinket she'd seen me admire in an empty mason jar in the back of my cupboard. It had taken me weeks to find it but when I had, late one night in pajamas and slippers, looking for a snack, I felt like I'd been given something magical. More than the trinket, she'd given me the gift of amazement.

I looked down at the seeds, shaking them in their paper packets to hear their satisfying rattle, and felt that same feeling now. What if, I thought, I tried to amaze a few people today?

I carried my cup and the seeds back inside and made some plans. I'd baked a batch of muffins the day before, full of poppy seeds and lemon. I put a few in an old cookie tin and tied a ribbon around it. I had a neighbor up the street whom I'd seen in the library a few days before. They were in the last semester of their degree and they'd been sitting with a tall stack of books and reams of notes all around them. I tucked a note in the tin: *Study snacks,* it said.

A few minutes later, I snuck the tin onto their front porch and ducked down the street toward the shops and café on the corner. I noticed a parking meter timed out in front of the grocery and slipped a few coins in from my pocket. I bought a small bouquet of daisies and daffodils and carried them into the bookstore. There was a tall shelf of historical fiction in the back and I slipped the flowers into a gap at the end of a row. I left a note there too; it just said, *For you.*

I walked through the park and picked up a few pieces of litter and left a quarter in the feed dispenser for the ducks. A dad with two little ones was juggling juice boxes, and I stopped for a second to help tie a shoe and open a pack of crackers. I held a door, I retrieved a dropped pencil, I took a picture of a dog sitting outside a shop and sent it to a friend I hadn't heard from in a while. I pointed a delivery man in the right direction. I lobbed an errant ball back into the schoolyard. I just smiled and slowed down. I thought that rushing was likely contagious and moving with some calm and ease was a way to help.

On my way back home, I stopped at the mailbox of the house across the street and slipped in a package of toy mice stuffed with catnip. The Siamese watched me from her spot on the back of the sofa. She stopped her bath and treated me to a quick flick of her tail.

Back in my own place, I laid out some newspapers on the kitchen table and got ready to plant my flower seeds. I'd stopped at a little art shop and bought some bright paints and tiny brushes. I dusted off the pots and brightened them up with the paints, sketching out designs and patterns as I went. I spooned potting mix in and sowed a few from each packet into the soil, thinking about how they would look when bloomed. Three small rainbows in terra-cotta. I watered them gently from the tap and set them out in saucers back on the front stoop. I'd painted a message on with my brushes and I turned them out to the street so my gift giver could read it when they passed by.

They said, "Thank you, friend."

Sweet dreams.

TEN IDEAS FOR
SIMPLE ACTS OF KINDNESS

· · · · ·

1. Leave a kind review for a business you enjoy.
2. Bring your neighbor's trash cans back up after garbage pickup.
3. Send a warmhearted text to a friend you haven't seen in a while.
4. Babysit for a parent in need of a night out.
5. When someone gives you great customer service, seek out their manager and pass on some praise.
6. Learn people's names and take time to say hello.
7. Keep an extra umbrella in your desk or bag so you can lend it out when it rains.
8. Don't look at your phone when you are in the company of others.
9. Leave unused coupons next to their corresponding products in the grocery store.
10. Tend to your own well-being. This is the highest form of charity.

Fireflies on a Summer Night

hildren are born believing in magic.

As I grew, I persisted in that believing. Adults tried to tell me magic wasn't real, that it was only something that happened in stories, but to me there were so many signs of it everywhere that it seemed like the adults were only trying to convince themselves. After all, what about when you slipped your finger into the coin return on a pay phone and found a quarter? What about when you opened a book to just the right page and your eyes fell on just the right word or drawing? What about when you found a stone that fit into your palm and hugged exactly around the curve of your thumb? And if magic wasn't real, then what about fireflies?

I would wait for them on summer nights, watching from the steps of the back deck or my bedroom window, and when they came, I thought they might be coming for me. Could we speak to each other— them in their language of slow-blinking glimmers, me in mine of quiet wonder? I'd step out in dewy grass and watch and wait. I never tried to seal them into jars, knowing even then that nobody likes to be boxed in. Instead I might reach out a hand and see if one wanted to rest on it for a moment. And when one did, when they stayed and blinked at me for a minute or so, I would wonder, *How is this not magic?*

I guess I persist in believing, even now that I'm all grown up. I still see it everywhere. What about when you're walking on the sidewalk and catch the eye of a stranger riding on a bus and you both hold on to each other's gaze for as long as you're in sight? What about when you step into your favorite café on a blustery, chilly day and find there's just one plate left of exactly what you were craving? What about when you learn that the iron in your blood was born in the belly of a star before the earth even was? And have you ever jumped into a lake on a hot summer day and, while you're completely surrounded by water, forgotten every other moment of your life? Go on, keep telling me how magic just happens in books.

Tonight was just the sort of evening when fireflies would be thick in the trees, so I thought I might go searching for them. I slipped sandals onto my bare feet and quietly closed the door behind me. Where should I look? In the garden? In the cluster of trees behind the shed? No, in the park. *Tonight, they'll be in the park*, I thought. I strode down the driveway, the air still hot from the day, and slipped down the street. Some houses had lights on inside, the top of a head and the edge of a book visible under the glow of a reading lamp. Some were quiet and dark, everyone already in bed. Days in the sun always meant good sleep. And a few houses had porches with dogs lying on the warm wooden boards, a neighbor or two sitting on a swing enjoying the night air. I raised a hand, answering the low calls of "Evening."

In the park, I circled slowly through the paths, smiled at an older lady, sitting with her gray-faced dog on a bench, gave some privacy to

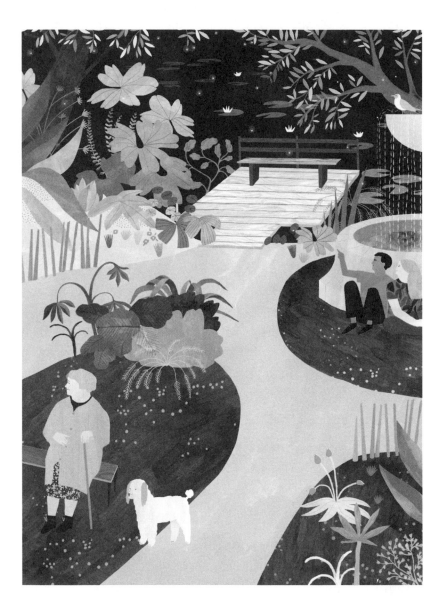

a couple cuddled up by the fountain, and made my way toward the edge of the pond. There was a tiny pier stretching out into water and I padded down it to the bench at the very end. The air was thick with the sound of frogs and night breezes and insects buzzing.

On the other side of the lake I saw them. Lighting up around the stems of hostas and flashing in front of the trunks of tall maples. I stood up and walked to the railing, leaning my elbows on the wood parapet. They glowed. They glimmered. Have you ever noticed how many very nice words for describing the effects of light on the world around us start with the letters *g* and *l*? Glint, glimmer, gleam. Gloss, glisten, glaze, and maybe the best one, gloaming. It was well past the gloaming now. Full dark was around me. I put my chin in my hand and just watched them. I'd heard once that there are mile-long stretches on the Nile where the fireflies all blink in unison. Can you imagine? How bright and then how dark and how much like language that must feel. They call that emergence. When order emerges from chaos. Maybe it was just another way to say magic.

After a while I made my way back down the wooden planks of the pier, back past the fountain, past the circle paths and benches and back down the streets of my neighborhood. In a neighbor's yard I saw the flames of a bonfire, a circle of chairs pulled up and friends laughing and telling stories. On another night I might have joined them, but tonight I was happy to be alone. To listen smilingly to their voices and make my way to my own quiet house.

I closed the front gate behind me and sat a moment on my front porch. The night sky was clear and full of stars and the visible glow of Mars. I knew Mars would set an hour after midnight, and soon after,

Jupiter and Saturn would rise. Then on the cusp of dawn Venus would shine and faintly behind her would be Mercury. They could set and rise without me. I thought of the softness of my sheets, my pillow cool and sweet-scented from the moving night air, and I stood and made my way inside. I turned the lock on my door and took a slow deep breath. Next would be sleep and dreaming. More magic.

Sweet dreams.

Someplace Only We Know

As a teenager I had a fascination with the romance of summer evenings.

I'd hop down the front steps of my house and think, *Anything could happen tonight.* Likely, nothing much would. My friends and I would spend another night drinking coffee in a diner, watching a movie, or listening to music on someone's car stereo in the lot by the park, but still, I never lost the feeling that summer nights had an extra dose of magical possibility. It's that warm night air—it makes us less afraid. The winter keeps us inside, nested and resting. The summer pushes us out: "Go meet someone, make a friend, discover something," it says.

The feeling had stayed with me as an adult. I'd almost stayed in tonight. I'd stood in the kitchen rinsing my plate after dinner (pasta tossed with olive oil, the first few cherry tomatoes of the season and a handful of herbs from the window box) and looked out at the evening sky. I could continue to sketch in my notebook and listen to music—more of that sounded just fine. But then the wind shifted and I felt the touch of it on my face. The kitchen filled up with the scent of summer night air and I felt that same pull from when I was fifteen. "Come out . . . come see . . . who knows what you might find?"

A few minutes later, I was coasting on my bike through the streets of my neighborhood. The day had been hot and the air rushing over my skin felt cooling and just right. I didn't know where I was going, just kept pedaling. I stood up on my pedals and pushed my way up a hill, then soared giddily down the other side. I circled through the district of old Victorian homes and slowed down to nosily peek through the wrought iron gates. Some were hiding tidy English gardens with rows of evenly spaced delphinium plants. In others I spied overgrown wilderness slowly reclaiming abandoned yards. I liked the abandoned places the best. They seemed full of secrets and stories.

I rode into town and skimmed past corners of bustling street cafés. People were eating and drinking and telling stories. I stopped at a light and looked at a couple sharing a meal. I thought it might be their first date. They seemed a little tentative as they threw quick glimpses back and forth before offering each other a laugh and an earnest smile. *Ah, maybe the second date*, I thought. I pedaled into the park and racked my bike by the bookstall, now shuttered for the night. I bought a lemon ice from a man with a cart and sat by the path for a few minutes to eat it.

There was something sweet on the edge of my memory. Something about this park. Maybe it was the lemon ice on my tongue that brought it back. Had we eaten it that night? I closed my eyes for a moment: it had been deep summer, the cicadas had been singing. We'd parked our bikes over there, in the rack by the fountain.

I decided to further explore the memory and got to my feet, dropping my empty cup in the recycle can. I turned toward a path at the back edge of the park, feeling pulled down it. It was narrow, gravel at first, then it became wood chips before it turned to packed sandy earth under my feet.

We'd come here, down this path, having found it just walking and exploring. The path opened into a broad meadow with a row of tall close boxwoods along one side. I turned to look at them now. They made a thick wall of green branches and seemed to mark the end of the park but . . . no. There was a space, camouflaged in the evening twilight, no wider than my shoulders where you could slip through and step down, and yes. Here it was.

That night, we'd stepped through and found this place, a sunken garden. We'd stood with wide eyes and I'd laughed in a nervous giddy way. We thought we'd stumbled on a place that had never been found before. Isn't that the way when you're young? You feel like you are discovering and inventing everything as you go. Like no one's ever loved like this before or had their heart broken like yours, or a million other instances of growing up and becoming yourself.

I studied the stone pool, long and a little green, running along the line of trees, and a small mossy bench in the corner and a crumbling statue of a lady disappearing into ivy. My heart beat a bit faster remembering. We'd been like the couple at the café, tentative and a little timid. But we couldn't beat back the power of a summer night;

it won out over shyness. Had it been me to reach out first? To lean in? Or had it been . . . ? Hmmm.

On my way back home, I pedaled along with the gift of memory like a sweet taste left on the tongue, so glad I'd gone out tonight. On a summer night, anything might happen. I could find my way back to something forgotten, to a place only we knew.

Sweet dreams.

A Concert in the Park

I t was a sunny day in the middle of the week in the middle of the summer.

I'd gotten home from work and puttered around in the yard for a while, then cut a vase's worth of tiger lilies and set them on the table by the front door, pulling out one extra bloom and setting it into a bud vase to sit on my bedside table. I'd had a sweetheart years ago who always did this for me—a vase of flowers on the table and one blossom by the bed—and I'd found it to be so romantic and cheerful that I'd kept the habit for myself ever since. Romance and cheer are important, even when you're by yourself.

I poured myself a glass of iced tea and watched cars going past from the kitchen window. I got lost in my imagination for a moment, staring out at the traffic. One car going straight, another turning, and I stood wondering where they were going on this lovely summer afternoon. I had that flash of understanding that sometimes happens when we step outside our own perspectives: that every person is the main character of their own story and we move in and out of the frame of others' stories as supporting characters or background players but we never really know any story but our own.

I set my glass down and my gaze fell on the calendar stuck with a magnet to the side of the fridge. Weeks ago I'd written in today's block of space *Concert in the park! 6:00 p.m.* I looked at my watch and saw that it was a quarter till; I'd have just enough time to walk into town and find a spot on a bench by the stage.

I pulled my bag over my shoulder and tied my sneakers on and started in a brisk pace toward the park. It felt good to walk fast and feel the summer air skimming over my skin. I looked into front yards as I passed, noticing different flowers and ground cover and leafy green perennials. There was an old house on a corner just by the park that had giant stone planters on either side of the front walkway and I stopped a moment to appreciate the elephant ears growing on long slim stems, which were now several feet tall. Their leaves were arrow shaped and soft with bright veins and seemed impossibly big. I looked forward to seeing how high they would grow by September.

I circled past the pond and around to a sunken space shaped like a clamshell, with built-in benches and a stage covered with a canopy of thin wooden slats laced over by a climbing vine.

The band was already playing; a four-piece jazz band with drums, a stand-up bass, piano, and horn. The benches around me were filling up with a combination of families and couples and people like me, who came on purpose to listen, and others, who had by happy accident heard the music on their way out of work and walked over to enjoy. I leaned my back against the cool stone of the bench behind me and closed my eyes to listen. The music followed a few familiar paths that I recognized from the old jazz records I'd been listening to since I was a child, then veered off into unfamiliar patterns and rhythms and circled back and veered away again. I looked up at the stage and watched the piano player and the horn player. They were watching each other, sometimes nodding in agreement as if to say, "Yes, good idea, more of that." Every now and then, one of them would crack a sudden smile and laugh, and I realized that someone in the band had somehow just told a musical joke. They were speaking a language that was foreign to me and I couldn't translate it or say what the joke was, but what I could hear was beautiful nonetheless.

I watched a little boy a few rows in front of me. He was watching the bass player as she thumped up and down the neck of the instrument with confident, strong fingers. As the horn blew and the melody turned in spirals in the air, she spun her bass on its end pin and caught it again in time to pluck out the next bit of rhythm. The little boy clapped his hands and swung his legs in time with the music.

I thought of a moment when I'd felt something similar. A different kind of concert a few years before. It was in an old roomy theater with creaking wooden seats and an expansive ceiling full of symmetrical painted murals framed in moldings that were already a hundred years old. A friend had pulled a few strings for me, knowing that this particular concert was a moment I'd dreamed of. She'd gotten me a seat dead center in the very front row, and when the man had walked onstage and sat down with his cello I could have nearly reached out and touched him. I'd expected to be enthralled by his playing, to be enraptured by the acoustics produced in the old theater. What I hadn't counted on were the tears that slipped down my cheeks, the feeling of my breath being taken from my body, the way I almost couldn't keep track of the notes as they thrummed through my chest. I'd gulped and pressed my hand over my heart and sat still so as to not break the spell while he played. I'd never had an experience quite like that before. This man hadn't just been speaking a language I didn't know; he seemed himself to have come from a different planet and was showing us what language was like on the other side of the cosmos.

Not everyone could make music like that, in fact only a few in every generation can, but that didn't diminish the joy of this simple concert in the park or the power of a string of notes to cut through thought and make us present. There was a clarinet player somewhere in my neighborhood whom I heard sometimes when I was out for a walk, the music coming from an open window in an upstairs room. The playing was sometimes squeaky and halting, but it was also patient and persistent and I was always glad to hear it. It made me think back to my own days in school band. I joked sometimes that I had played eighth chair flute even though there were only five of us. The truth was that because it hadn't come quickly to me, I'd given up. In my immature brain I figured that if I couldn't be the best, I would quit. The folly of youth. I was glad that years had passed and given me their wisdom, that now I could see that I didn't have to be the best, that there was a whole lot of joy and meaning and learning to be had in the act of simply playing.

I hoped the boy swinging his legs and clapping along to the music would be a bit wiser than I had when his turn for school band came around, though I reminded myself, everyone has their own journey to understanding. Everyone has their own story to tell.

Sweet dreams.

Summer Nights

We swam all day.

We ran down the dock, our wet feet slapping on the sun-bleached boards, and made sloppy dives and cannonballs into the lake. We tooled around on paddleboards and kayaks. We floated lazily on inner tubes, fingers trailing in the water. We talked. We sang along to the radio and told jokes and cracked each other up. Then we pulled ourselves up onto lounge chairs, jammed straw hats over our faces, stretched out and fell asleep in the hot summer sun. When we woke, we raided the coolers for cold drinks, ate chips and salsa, and jumped back into the lake, splashing water onto our magazines and paperback books.

When the sun tipped into the afternoon sky, we pulled shorts and tank tops over our swimsuits and padded into the house to make a big summer feast of a dinner. The gardens were overflowing and the farmers market stalls had been too tempting to resist that week, so the house was full of summer vegetables and fresh fruits. We handed two dozen ears of corn to a few of our group who carried them out to the back porch to shuck the fresh husks off into brown paper bags. We lit the barbecue and laid out thick slices of seasoned eggplant and squash and tiny new potatoes. We marinated portobello mushrooms and added them, sizzling, to the grill.

My Italian grandma taught me that when vegetables are in their peak season, as all of ours were, you should serve them simply with good olive oil, garlic, a bit of sea salt, and an herb or two. Since we had picked a huge bowl of green beans from the garden that morning, I made them into an *insalata di fagiolini* per my grandma's recipe—adding in lots of fresh mint and a splash of tart vinegar. And as the vegetables were coming off the grill, I cut thick slices of farm bread, two loaves at least, and set them out on the grill to crisp. I had a mountain of ripe avocados to go with them and I carefully halved and pitted them. You know that satisfying feeling when you slide your knife through an avocado and twist the halves apart and know before you've even seen the inside that it is perfectly ripe, green and soft and without a bruise anywhere? I enjoyed it again and again as I set the toasts on a tray and scooped out healthy portions of the mashed fruit on top. I doused some with hot sauce and served up others with just a good sprinkle of salt and pepper.

As everyone gathered around the table, I laid out the trays of toast and bowls of the tangy crisp beans. There were grilled vegetables, fresh salads, hot sweet corn, and plates of homemade hummus, salsas, and herby pesto. We talked over each other, reached for dishes, passed them, and ate off each other's plates. We poured cold water into cups, dug beer out of the cooler, opened bottles of rosé and prosecco, and ate and ate and ate. As the sun started to sink behind the trees, we pushed our plates back and stayed at the table, talking, citronella candles lit to ward off summer bugs. Someone brought out bowls of fresh berries and a hot cobbler from the oven. "No!" we cried. "No more. We can't." But we found a way.

We carried our plates into the house and some kind soul started washing dishes. Another started to dry. We turned up the radio and sang as we tidied and wiped down the counters. I sneaked to my room and pulled on an old pair of lounge pants and a warm soft hoodie. My skin was sun kissed and chilled at the same time, and the fresh clothes felt so good. I washed my face, put on lip balm, found my flip-flops, and headed back out.

There was a fire now, and all the chairs had been pulled up around it. We propped up our feet and looked at the stars that were just starting to show. Fireflies were blinking in the trees, and a breeze brought the smell of the water into our noses. There is a feeling, on summer nights, when you look up at the sky and suddenly remember how old the universe is, how big it is, and how small and simple you are. It was a comfort to me to remember that I was small and that I may as well set aside my worries and grudges and take joy where I could find it. I looked around at the faces of my friends: the firelight shining in their eyes, all of us laughing and talking and making memories together. I was contented to be where I was, and grateful to be with them.

Leaning my head back against the old Adirondack chair, I took a deep breath of summer night air. Tonight, I would sleep, deep and peaceful.

Sweet dreams.

Avocado Toast Four Ways

. . . .

MAKES 2 SLICES

The lovely thing about avocado toast is that it can be just as delicious when it's simple as when it's fancied up. It can be a satisfying quick breakfast or made into the star of the show at lunch or dinner. Be sure to start with good bread, something sturdy to hold all that mashed deliciousness. I love sourdough or a seedy loaf with swirls of pumpernickel or rye.

2 slices good-quality bread, thickly sliced

1 ripe avocado, pitted, peeled, and sliced

PLAIN AND SIMPLE TOAST

Salt and pepper, to taste

SMOKY AND TANGY MEXICAN TOAST

Chipotle hot sauce (Tabasco has a good one!), to taste

1/4 teaspoon Tajín seasoning, or to taste

KIMCHI SESAME TOAST

1/2 cup kimchi

2 tablespoons toasted sesame seeds

SALAD-TOPPED TOAST

1 cup loosely packed arugula

1 tablespoon extra virgin olive oil

1 teaspoon fresh lemon juice

Toast the bread.

Spoon half the avocado onto each slice of bread and mash it lightly with a fork.

To make the Plain and Simple Toast: Sprinkle salt and pepper evenly over the avocado, to taste.

To make the Smoky and Tangy Mexican Toast: Sprinkle the hot sauce and Tajín evenly over the avocado, to taste. Tajín seasoning is a lovely mix of chili peppers, salt, and lime. It's quite tangy, so taste a bit on your finger before you sprinkle.

To make the Kimchi Sesame Toast: Layer 1/4 cup of kimchi onto each slice of toast over the avocado and top with the sesame seeds. If you have only raw or untoasted sesame seeds, try toasting them in a dry pan over low heat for a minute or so, shaking the pan frequently. When they start to smell toasty and nutty and have a bit of light brown color, take them off the heat and use immediately. Freshly toasted sesame seeds have an amazing flavor and are a great addition to simple green salads, rice or noodle bowls, and, of course, avocado toast.

To make the Salad-Topped Toast: Place the arugula in a medium bowl. Drizzle with the olive oil and lemon juice. Toss until the arugula is evenly coated. Divide the arugula evenly among the pieces of toast, balancing as much as you can on top of the avocado.

Off the Beaten Path

I've always been one to turn off the main roads and go looking for someplace I've never been before.

Maybe I'm hoping to be surprised by something, to see a hidden ruin rising out of a clump of trees or to stumble across a waterfall where I'd never known there to be one. Most times I find more woods, more fields, more old houses tumbling down on forgotten farmland, but even those things are pretty magical. Sometimes I spot old tree houses still holding their own in the branches of a tall tree. I like to think about who climbed the planks tacked into its bark, who played pretend from the tiny house above, and where they might be today. I wonder if they sometimes stop and remember the way the wood felt under their fingers as they climbed.

Today was the perfect day for exploring, with blue skies and warm summer air coming in through the open car windows. I stopped at a shady intersection and looked up and down the rutted dirt road. I looked left and turned, bits of gravel skittering out from under my tires. The roads were a bit rough and hilly, crisscrossed constantly by chipmunks and squirrels, so I went slowly and stopped every now and then to get a better look into a field or grove of trees. I turned another corner and stopped short so a rafter of turkeys could peck and strut and flap their way across the road.

I kept driving, feeling a bit lost and enjoying it. I had no place to be, so wherever I was, it was just right. The hills smoothed out into broader flattened fields, and I saw a few silos in the distance, then a few busy farms, tractors and thrashers moving over the land.

Beyond the meadows of corn and wheat, there was a patch of land covered with a bright purple haze. I tipped my face toward the window and breathed in the sweet smell of fresh growing lavender. Farther down the road I saw a drive that turned toward the purple fields and at its entrance a sign saying they were open and happy to have visitors.

I'd never seen so many lavender plants in one place: They covered the fields on either side of the drive in neat, evenly spaced rows. They surrounded a small house and parking lot and continued as far back as I could see into the acres beyond. I parked in the small lot and left my windows down with the hopes that the flowery scent in the air would settle into my car. And then I just walked for a while, through the rows of plants, stopping now and then to press my hand into the shrubby stems and feel their short green leaves, which looked a bit like rosemary. Their bright purple flowered heads left my skin scented with the clean, almost minty aroma that reminded me of the soap in my shower but was a thousand times more potent and astonishing. I thought that if I had been a healer living centuries before and had stumbled upon these plants for the first time, I would immediately have recognized them as medicine.

I followed a gravel path that circled through the fields and saw a few small structures and cleared spaces to explore. There was a humble shop built from an old shed, filled with shelves of homemade soaps and satchels stuffed with tiny purple grains. There were bottles of potent essential oil that the man behind the counter proudly told me they distilled themselves, along with glass jars of lavender water to spray on linens and laundry, and candles speckled with green-and-purple flecks of the plant. I gathered a small collection of items, including a precious tiny bottle of the oil, and paid my dollars, which went into an old tin box under the counter.

The man pointed farther down the path and invited me to keep wandering. I thanked him and took him up on the offer. Soon there was another shed, this one with every inch of wall space dedicated to drying lavender. It hung in overlapping bundles—heads down and stems in the air. There were hundreds of bouquets and the air inside was hot and thick with the scent. I stood and let it settle over me. Breathing it in, I felt calm and relaxed and thought that I had never been in a spa that smelled this good. Sometimes modern luxuries just can't re-create what nature produces so prolifically.

Outside the drying shed was a tall copper still and, beside it, a small gray-haired woman was attaching a coiled tube to the boiler. She smiled up at me and asked if I knew how they turned their fields of lavender into the oil they sold in their shop. I said that I didn't but was happy to learn. She pulled off thick work gloves and reached into a basket to bring out a handful of fresh lavender stalks. She told me she'd cut them that morning, close to the flower head without much stem; that's the process that produces the best quality oil. As she told me the story of distillation, how the kettle is packed full of lavender and steamed slowly to extract the oil, she walked me around the still and we squatted down together to see where oil separates from the vapor and is caught in a glass bottle. I guessed she'd given this same talk hundreds if not thousands of times before, but she still seemed excited and proud to share the secrets of the process. Afterward, she tilted her head forward, as if to suggest there was more to find farther down the path.

I'd set out today to explore, guessing that I'd likely see just the usual fields and forests, but hoping I might come across something unexpected. I reminded myself how sweet it is to be surprised, how good to wander off the beaten path.

Sweet dreams.

A Letter in an Envelope

aybe it was in second grade, or maybe third, but we'd read a book about pen pals, featuring a little girl from Portugal and a little boy from Japan.

They sent letters back and forth, talking about their families and pets and schools. There'd been an illustration of each of them waiting for the mail to come, eager to hear again from a friend on the other side of the world. It created a bit of a craze for letter writing in my class, and our teacher presented us with a list of names and addresses of children in a class in Poland who were keen on being pen pals. I'd drawn the name of a girl named Anna and dutifully set out to write her a letter. I don't remember much now about what I wrote her or what she wrote me, but I do remember the excitement of finding her letter in my mailbox, the green paper of the envelope and the exotic look of her handwriting. I remember her number fours and how she'd inked out her *j*'s and *f*'s.

While Anna and I lost touch among the shifting responsibilities of elementary school, I never stopped writing letters and mailing them off to friends, flowers pressed into their pages, drawings of birds and trees haphazardly sketched across their envelopes, sometimes just a postcard with a joke written hastily, sometimes many pages needing extra stamps and strips of tape to hold them closed. I had bundles of letters I'd received in return—tied with scraps of ribbon and bits of twine—in a long squat box tucked under my bed. Sometimes on a rainy day, I'd dig out a pack to see what we were all talking about ten years ago.

I'd been thinking about those letters under the bed this morning when I heard the flap and clatter of my mail slot. I'd been spreading peanut butter onto a thick slice of toast for breakfast. I carried the handful of envelopes and mailers back to my kitchen table, and when I spotted the corner of an envelope, pale blue with a hand-drawn heart, I felt that same excitement that the boy from Japan and the girl from Portugal must have felt. It was a little square envelope with my name written in tiny neat script and stickers of flowers sealing it shut. I propped it up against my glass of grapefruit juice and sat down to finish my toast. I like waiting a bit to open a letter, letting the antici- pation build, plus I didn't want to get peanut butter on that pretty blue paper. I took my time, working my way through my toast and juice and a lovely ripe banana, tidying up my plates and washing my hands be- fore I carried the letter to a sunny spot on the back porch where I could look out at the growing garden as I read.

The letter was from a childhood friend; we'd grown up on the same street but now lived far apart. Many people who rarely see each other write long letters to catch up, updates on work and love and family, and certainly that is all useful and welcome information, but my friend and I didn't send those kinds of letters to each other. We sent little collections of interesting things, whatever seemed curious to us at the time of sending.

This time, inside the envelope I found a list of books she'd read in the past month with a series of hand-drawn stars beside each one to show what she'd thought, a recipe on an index card for a curry dish her neighbor made, a ticket stub from a play she'd seen with a line that had stuck with her written on the back, a note from her little boy about summer camp, and a stick of gum, the kind I had loved to chew in high school. I opened the foil and chewed it right there on the porch as I looked back through the little stash of finds. There were a couple of books on her list that I had also read and I thought about how I'd have ranked them. I realized I had all the ingredients for the curry dish and figured that evening's dinner was now sorted out. I remembered some stories from our own days at summer camp and thought I might write some out for my reply.

I stepped back inside and flipped through my stationery box. There was paper in lots of sizes and shades, postcards bought on faraway travels or just from the corner store, and a stack of old photos. I'd been collecting them for ages, some from old albums in the attic and some found here and there, at garage sales and flea markets. I sometimes held an old photo, a very old one, and wondered if it was the last image left of that person. They'd had a whole life somewhere, loves and losses, favorite songs and sworn enemies, and it felt like

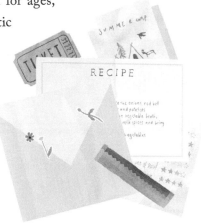

taking a moment to look at them gave them a breath of life again. I shuffled through them and pulled out a Polaroid from the sixties of a little boy sitting on a terribly patterned sofa with his grandma, and another, older, from the thirties, of two girls in dresses standing in front of a clapboard front porch. On the strip of space under the Polaroid I wrote "Stuff a date with almond butter, or mint leaves . . . but not both." On the back of the picture of the girls I wrote a note for my friend's son. It said, "Ask your mom about the camp talent show. Does she still tap dance?" I smiled at the memory and wondered if it would make the little boy laugh. I added in a scrap I'd cut out from the police blotter of the local paper about a woman who'd been stealing flowers from her neighbor's yard, underlining the words SUSPECT HAS NOT BEEN APPREHENDED. Lastly, I jotted down a few lines about the lecture I went to at the library that week—a talk about grafting apple trees. "The scion," I explained, was the part being grafted. "The rootstock," I told her, was its new home.

I bundled it all into an envelope and sealed it with red wax, pressing a star-shaped stamp into it. A letter received and a letter written. Wondering if my friend would remember the story from grade school, I wrote across the envelope, "From Japan to Portugal."

Sweet dreams.

At the Summer Fair

As kids, we always went during the day.

We'd ride the rides and play the games, eat pretzels with lines of yellow mustard squeezed on top and blue snow cones that stained our lips. We didn't mind the heat and ran from one booth to another, calling out to each other about where to go next. At some point we'd be rounded up and taken home, dusty and exhausted and still chattering about all the things we'd seen and done.

Now as grown-ups we like to go in the late afternoon, as the sun is sinking behind the trees—the hottest part of the day behind us and the breeze of evening starting to break through the midsummer air.

Today, we set out from home hand in hand and made our way toward the sound of the fair in the distance. In my memory the fairgrounds were huge, paths you could get lost in and always a corner of the park that you hadn't explored. But now I saw that it had only ever been the green space of the city park and the gravel lot beside it, with a row of artists' booths stretching down the riverfront.

All along the edges of the fairground were tall wooden bins filled by a local orchard with the ripe stone fruits of the season. Peaches and plums and nectarines and tiny yellow-orange apricots were heaped in sweet-smelling mounds. The fruit was so abundant at this point in the summer and the orchard so generous that you could just help yourself to anything that sounded good. Plums are my favorite, but if they aren't perfectly ripe, they can be terribly sour and hard to get your teeth through.

We stopped to survey the offerings and I found a couple small but soft and ripe-smelling plums. They had a frosted shimmer on their skins, with deep purple underneath. I slipped them into my pocket to eat later, maybe after a short stay in the fridge. It made me think suddenly of that brief lovely poem by William Carlos Williams about plums in the icebox.

We linked hands again and stepped into the heart of the fair. Kids ran and chased; bunches of friends strolled on the midway; a teddy bear clamped under an arm, won at a booth somewhere along the way. The people watching was excellent: here was an older couple watching from a bench, canes propped beside and a huge bag of popcorn between them, their hands bumping together as they reached in for another mouthful. Here was a grunt of teens (that is the collective noun for teenagers, a grunt or alternatively an attitude of teens), boastful and merrily loud after a couple months of running free from school, holding court by the Ferris wheel. Here were four women who looked so much alike they must be sisters, each with long dark hair and bright shades of lipstick, having a good gossip, while an occasional kid would run up to ask for a dollar or hand over a cast-off sweater. Lucky children, I thought, when you can turn as easily to an aunt as to your mom to have your shoelace tied. They won't know till they're older how sweet that is.

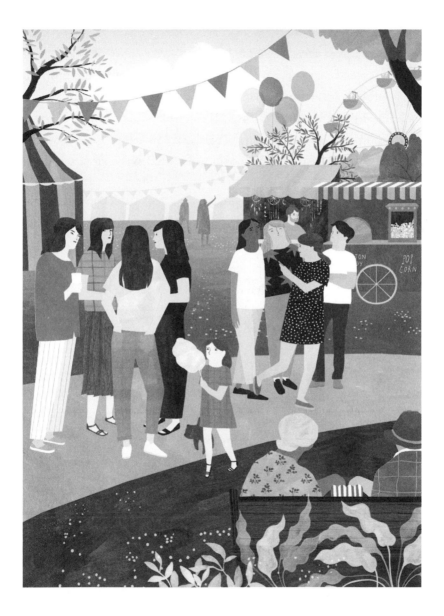

We rode the Ferris wheel lots back when we were teenagers ourselves. We didn't need any teddy bears and we weren't yet ready to sit on a bench and eat popcorn, so we walked past all of that and down to the booths of art and handmade things by the river. We went slowly, looking at silver rings set with polished stones, watercolors of some local landmarks, soaps and salves (I bought something good for mosquito bites), tiny hand-bound books you could write stories in, and rows and rows of ceramics.

I'm a sucker for teacups and coffee mugs—however many I've got, I'd always like one more. As I was looking, I got a little squeeze from the hand I was holding, which I knew meant go on, pick out a good one. I found a squat little cup, the glaze a smooth bluish green, with a broad spot at the top of the handle to rest your thumb. It was paid for, and I watched as it was wrapped up in yesterday's newspaper and tucked into my bag for tomorrow morning's tea. *I'll use it with my plums*, I thought.

The sunlight was going and the tall streetlamps were coming on around us. We could turn home, and soon we would, but maybe we'd just walk a bit farther along the river first. After all, in the course of a year, these summer nights were few and should be savored. *Let's walk a bit farther.*

Sweet dreams.

Stargazing in the Woods

T here is a kind of quiet out in the woods that is different from the quiet of a city or neighborhood street.

Because the woods aren't actually quiet. There are layers of sound coming down from the branches as birds call and leaves rustle together. There are layers of sound coming up from the forest floor as chipmunks race and deer take sure-footed steps and insects click and buzz. No, the quiet that happens in the woods isn't in the woods; it's in us when we are there. That's what we came for, the quiet that settles deep in the bones after a few days away from everything else, even the things we loved. Sometimes we need space from them too.

We made a campsite in a clearing under tall pines, whose needles made a thick carpet for our tent. Around the grove of trees there were pockets of open space, fields where we could walk or watch animals as they moved through their daily routines. Beyond them, far in the distance, we could see a rising peak of something that was more than a hill but not quite a mountain. We dug out a place for a fire and rolled out our sleeping bags, organized our food, and settled camp chairs in the best spot for watching sunsets. Afterward, we wandered for a bit and found a fast-moving stream, where I trailed my fingers through the water, then explored a well-worn path down to the lake, along the way gathering a few smooth flat stones that we would skip with varying levels of success across its surface.

At night we watched fireflies. They were like moving constellations and I found shapes in them the same way I'd found shapes in the clouds during the day. All the while, the quiet was settling deeper into my system. I was finding my focus again. Sometimes in the busy blur of work and home and my to-do list, my mind struggles to stay on the path I carve out for it. I can't sustain my attention, and it's led me to forget things and leave projects half finished. Out here, however, I noticed that I could just listen to the morning song of the birds or watch the minnows swimming circles around my ankles in the lake and my senses stayed where I put them. It hadn't happened all at once, but it had happened.

Tomorrow we would pack up and go back. I would be ready to go back then, but for tonight I wanted to go a bit further into the quiet and spend some time all by myself. We both did. As good as togetherness is, being separate has its own appeal, so I pulled on my hiking boots and stepped out onto a trail to find a place to look at the stars.

It was a cloudless night, and I found my way easily as I cleared the line of trees at the edge of our campsite. There was a spot I'd been to a few times during the week. It was a bit higher up on a slope with a flat rock just big enough for me to stretch out on. I'd gone before to look down at the lake and across to the tops of trees on its far side, though tonight I meant only to look up. It took a few minutes to get there, and as I walked I felt the path under my feet. It seemed I'd gotten more sensitive to finding the right way to step, the places where I could solidly land my boots. It's something I forgot sometimes, that we get better at what we do habitually, whether it's a hike in the woods, learning a new language, or even just being patient when something goes awry. It was something my mother used to recite, "Say a kind word today and it will come even easier tomorrow."

I'd brought an old plaid blanket and when I reached my spot, I flung it out and let it ripple over the flat rock, then stretched out, tucked my hands behind my head, and crossed one ankle over the other in a posture of sincere stargazing. The stars were so bright, it took my breath away. I almost couldn't bear to blink. I was used to a night sky that shared its space with so many streetlights and billboards and buildings that the stars were just a dim part of the background, but out here they were the entire sky. They were astonishingly brilliant and though they were so far away, they felt nearly touchable.

I thought of where I was on this rock, in this stretch of forest, and I let my perspective expand. I zoomed out, taking in more space. I thought of the cities around me, then the borders of countries, the immense spread of oceans. I thought of myself like a tiny spark of light, along with all the billions of other sparks, lighting up our small blue dot. I kept zooming out thinking about planets I'd learned to name in elementary school, suspended in space around me. The rings of Saturn, Neptune's dark spot, Jupiter with his fifty-three moons. I stretched my thoughts further, to space beyond what we could see with telescopes or predict with equations, figuring that out past all of it there wasn't likely to be a big brick wall but instead more and more endless expanse. I slowly started to zoom back in.

I pulled my thoughts back through space, back from the planets and sun, back to our spot in the universe. I zoomed in tighter to see the shape of the continent, the formations and lakes and mountain chains around me. I zoomed right down to my rock and back into my body. I felt my breath moving through my nostrils and the relaxed slow beat of my heart. I felt the weight of my limbs and the touch of my clothes.

Somewhere along the way, my perspective had realigned. I'd come for quiet, and I'd found it, but beyond that I was resettled in my body and my heart, remembering who I was and what mattered to me. I was ready to go back.

Sweet dreams.

The quiet that happens

in the woods isn't

in the woods; it's in us

when we are there.

The Dog Days of Summer

We'd woken nose to nose, as usual.

We lay still for a while, blinking at each other, shifting out of the last dream of the morning and listening to the birds singing in the branches. Then, she started to wag her tail, happy energetic thumps that shook the bed, and I couldn't help but laugh. My dog wakes up happy every day.

That day she had every right to be. I was all hers and we had plans to do some favorite things. She jumped out of bed and I followed, still a little sleepy, rubbing my eyes and taking deep breaths of morning air.

We stepped outside together and while she nosed through the grass and attended to her morning toilette, I stood still and just looked into the branches of the oak trees. Squirrels were tracing routes through the limbs, carrying breakfast in their bulging cheeks; robins and one tall blue jay were flitting about in the leaves. Morning business. I stooped near the edge of the vegetable patch to absentmindedly pull a few stray weeds from around my tomato plants. The grass was dewy; it felt cool on my feet and the plants sparkled. I lifted a broad prickly leaf in the garden and underneath found a perfect cucumber that I twisted off the vine.

I stood and took a lungful of that warm summer morning air,

which smelled so richly of green growing things and lush black earth. Have you ever been carried back in time by a scent? In an instant, I remembered a camping trip when I was a child, maybe five or six. We'd stayed in a tiny cabin and cooked outside as the sun set. My father had entertained us with a story he'd started on the first night and added onto each evening with twists and turns, bandits and princesses and buried treasure.

I thought also of the good dogs we'd had as I was growing up; they'd taught me how to be gentle, how to play, and the goodness that comes from caring for someone else.

I patted my hand against my thigh to call my dog. She padded over, nose damp from poking through the dewy plants, and sniffed at the vegetables I'd picked. "Breakfast then?" I asked. She ran for the door. This is part of our routine each morning; when we come back in from the garden, she races as fast as she can to the kitchen and sits, tail drumming against the cabinet, waiting for her treat.

When I first brought her home and we were still getting to know each other, I used to just hand it to her and she would politely take it and carry it under the kitchen table to eat. But after a few weeks, when she'd gotten more comfortable and was letting me see more of who she was, she would take the treat and attempt to toss it to herself in the air. I imagine she was trying to teach me, to show me that even a snack could be fun, that everything can be play. And she'd trained me well.

That morning, when I caught up with her in the kitchen and asked if she was sure she wanted a treat (here there was more tail thumping and her eyes opened as wide as they could), I took a biscuit from her jar on the counter and darted my hand left and right, sending her in excited circles. Finally I tossed it into the air and she expertly clicked her teeth around it.

"Right," I said, patting her head and turning to the coffeepot. "Let's see about today."

I made my coffee, filled her bowl with kibble, and dropped a couple slices of seedy bread into the toaster. I sliced the cucumber, and when the toast popped up, I spread it thick with hummus. I layered on the cucumber, then sprinkled on salt and pepper and some sprouts from a jar on the windowsill. My girl was crunching away and I dropped into the chair closest to her so we could breakfast together. In between bites, I said casually, "So I was thinking . . . dog park?" She stopped with her mouth full and looked at me, not sure if she'd heard me right. I said it again. "Dog park?" She jumped, she danced, she wriggled up beside me to have her back scratched and patted. When dogs are happy, their instinct is to share it. For me this is proof enough that the universe bends toward kindness.

Now that the words had been spoken, she was eager to go. Another lesson from her to me: when you know what you want, go get it. We got dressed, me in a sundress and sandals, her in her harness and neckerchief, which proclaimed, if her goofy smile wasn't enough to do so, that she was happy to be petted. I jingled the keys and we raced to the car. With the window down enough so that she could feel the wind in her ears and smell all the good scents of the neighborhood, we drove off. Soon we were turning into the gravel lot beside the park and I watched her dipping her head eagerly side to side, looking between the trees, trying to see through the fence who was there. Old buddies? New friends?

Inside the park and off her leash, she dashed about, sniffing at the other dogs, barking and bowing to get a game going. There were a few old-timers, with sweet white faces, lying about and watching the younger ones chase. There were scrappy little dogs bossing the group and running fast on stilty legs, fluffy slower dogs dipping back and forth between the play and the comfort of Mom's or Dad's ankles. I sat on a bench in a shady corner and watched them all. It made my heart shine to see my girl confident and comfortable, at ease in her life.

She was already a few years old when she'd come to live with me and I remembered her uncertain face on the drive home from the shelter. I'd told her that her last bad day was yesterday, that from now on she was safe and her whole life would be about play and naps and walks and whatever else she liked, but that's something you have to show not tell. By now I'd shown her, and she trusted her life.

The games were winding down, the doggies were getting pleasantly worn out, and leashes were being clicked onto collars. My girl found me and I poured the water from my bottle into a bowl I'd brought. She took a good long drink and we got back in the car. I wanted to treat her all day, so I thought next we'd stop by her favorite pet shop and pick out a new toy. Then later a long walk and a nap on the shady back porch. After dinner I'd throw a ball for her until she got tired. I wouldn't make her have a bath till tomorrow. Eventually we'd climb back into bed. She'd turn around three times, plop down and let out that little doggy huff, and we would sleep.

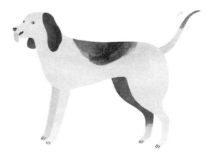

Sweet dreams.

When dogs are happy,

their instinct is to share it.

For me this is proof enough

that the universe bends

toward kindness.

LOVING-KINDNESS MEDITATION

. . . . .

Think of it like this: you have kindness and compassion in you (everybody does) but sometimes it's packed in a random box in your basement, and if you need it you might not be able to get your hands on it in a hurry. Loving-kindness Meditation (also called Metta Meditation) helps you dig it out, dust it off, and keep it in your front pocket. When you bump into someone who needs it, you can offer it up easily with plenty to spare. This meditation is also a balm for rough days; it soothes a heavy spirit and leaves you simply feeling better about the world.

Start by getting comfortable. More than with any other style of meditation, a comfortable posture is important here. I want you to be at ease in your body so you can focus completely on warming up your heart. Sit in a comfy chair or lie down somewhere nice. You can use a bolster under your knees to make it that much sweeter.

Take a slow breath in through your nose and sigh it out of your mouth. Then, start to breathe naturally and for a minute or so, just point your attention at your breath, as it comes in and goes out.

Now you need to remember what loving-kindness feels like in your body, because there is a physical sensation that goes along with love and loving. There is probably a person in your life with whom, when you see them or when you just think of them, you feel an uncomplicated heart-to-heart feeling—a pure desire for them to be well and happy. (And it's just fine if that person is your dog.) Spend a few minutes wishing that person well. With all the love in your heart, send them hopes for health and happiness.

Say in your head, "May they be happy. May they know real peace and harmony. May they feel safe. May they come out of their suffering."

Keep your attention there, on how loving feels, for a few moments. You're opening the well of loving-kindness in your heart, and once it's open, you can dip down and draw out more as needed. You can let it overflow. If it hasn't been open in a while and the cover has rusted a bit, well . . . be patient. It's only a matter of time and practice.

Without letting that light go out, reach out with your mind for another person. Someone who is peripheral to your life, whose happiness you might not have thought of much before. With the same earnestness and openhearted desire for their well-being, wish them well.

Say in your head, "May they be happy. May they know real peace and harmony. May they feel safe. May they come out of their suffering."

Hold on to the idea of them feeling good and safe and happy for a moment. If you can picture things in your head, picture how their face might look if they were truly at peace: worry lines relaxed and eyes clear and bright.

Without letting that light go out, reach out for one more person with your mind. This time, let it be someone whom you find quite difficult to wish well. Maybe in the past you've wished the exact opposite. But listen: when we hold bitterness for someone else, we get the strongest dose of the poison in our own hearts and heads first. Likewise, when we draw up compassion and forgiveness for someone, we're the first to get the strongest dose of medicine. So source that clear loving-kindness, the stuff that bubbles up for your dog or your daughter or your sweetheart, and offer it up to this person.

And even if it will never change anything for them, and they will never know or care, say in your head, "May they be happy. May they know real peace and harmony. May they feel safe. May they come out of their suffering."

Don't let the lights go out. Let the medicine work in your system for a few moments; continue to dip into the well and let it spill through your every part and piece. When you feel settled and ready to move on, take another deep breath in through the nose and release a big exhale through your mouth.

Good.

In the Kitchen, During a Storm

I t was early evening and I was flipping through a case of old records.

Hmm. Billie Holiday? Ella? Oh, Chet Baker. That will do nicely. I slipped the album out of the sleeve and tilted the surface to the light, blowing the dust off before sliding it onto the turntable. I lifted the needle and let it touch down into the groove of the record, then leaned back in my chair and put my feet up. As I listened, I hummed along and, tucking one arm behind my head, looked out the window at the silver undersides of leaves on the trees in my back garden.

The wind was picking up. It had been a gray day, but still humid and hot. In the last hour or so I'd felt the temperature begin to drop. I stood and stepped barefoot through my back door and onto the still-warm stones of my patio. I took a deep breath to taste the air. Rain was coming.

There is a feeling of energy around a storm; at first it seems like it might be due to the relief of the cooling air, but then there is an excitement, a sense of potential that boosts you up and clears your head. I stood a while longer, looking out at the darkening sky and gripping the stones under my feet with my toes. I knew what I would do.

I stepped back into the house and walked through the rooms, cracking windows and lighting candles. I turned the music higher and stepped into the kitchen, where I hadn't spent much time for a few days because of the heat. I had a large window over my kitchen sink and a row of potted herbs stood on its sill. It was an old window, as it was an old house, so I had to

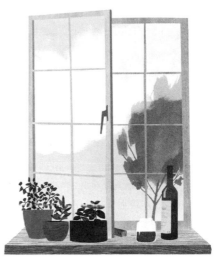

prop it open with a short wooden block to keep it from slamming shut. The breeze blew through my tiny herb garden, and I could smell basil and oregano.

I had a bottle of red wine open from the night before, and I reached into a cupboard for a jam jar to drink from. Sometimes I am fancy and use my best stemmed wineglasses, but often when I am home alone and just puttering about the kitchen, drinking from an old squat jam jar seems just about right. I pulled a wooden chopping board from a drawer and laid out my chef's knife and put a wide low skillet on the range. I was going to make spaghetti al pomodoro, the way I had been taught years ago in Italy. It was an incredibly simple dish that used only a few ingredients and came together in no time, but its tangy bright flavor took me straight back to afternoon meals around my family's table on the rocky southern Italian coast. I'd been a foreign exchange student and although I didn't possess of drop of Italian blood,

I felt that after a year walking her streets and learning her language and falling in love with her people, I had earned some Italian-ness. My host family had taken me in and loved me, laughed at my funny accent, and rolled their eyes at my overly independent American tendencies, but I'd become a member of the family. Years later, we were still close.

Lunch came at around 2:00 p.m. in Italy, and trudging home from school I would wonder what kind of pasta my host mother—Mamma— would be cooking that day. I'd take the stairs, four flights up, to our apartment, slip my house key into the lock, and crack the door just an inch. Then I'd stick my nose into the doorway and take a deep breath in.

Now, more or less a grown-up in my own home, I smiled at the memory and pulled together the ingredients for my dinner. I filmed the bottom of the pan with good olive oil and took a yellow onion from the pantry. Mamma had shown me many times that less was more in her cooking. That just because you have a whole onion, doesn't mean the dish needs a whole onion. I was a dutiful daughter and cut a third off the whole and sliced through the layers a few times. I slipped them into the pan and turned the heat to low. I just wanted to warm them through and give them a tiny bit of color. Back to the pantry for a can of whole peeled tomatoes, grown and packed just a few miles from where I had lived. Mamma passed them through an old-fashioned food mill in her kitchen, turning the crank slowly and letting the to- mato skins catch in the wire weave of the filter. It made a smooth sauce that slipped over the noodles and coated them. I tipped mine into a bowl and used my fingers to break them up a bit instead. I didn't tell Mamma this—everyone has their secrets. I added the tomatoes to the pan and poured salt into the palm of my hand to measure it, then dusted it down into the tomatoes and stirred. I kept the heat on the low end of medium and I pinched a few basil leaves from my pot by the window to toss whole into the sauce. The rain was falling now, and I pressed my palm to the sill to check if it was raining in; it wasn't, and I was glad. The smell of the grass and trees cooling in the rain was lovely.

I put a pot of water on the stove for the spaghetti and sipped from my jam jar. The record had stopped and I wandered back into the other room to turn it over. As I set the needle on the record, I saw a flash of lightning in the darkening sky. I waited, sitting back on my heels by the record player as the rumbling thunder grew louder. What a perfect night for pasta and wine.

My water was boiling, and I spun the spaghetti into the pot so it spread out and began to sink. Some people stand over the pot and test the noodles every few minutes or do some other nonsense about throwing pieces against the wall, but if you want properly cooked al dente pasta, it's simple. Buy good pasta made in Italy and cook it for the length of time it says on the package. They know what they're doing.

I set a place for myself where I could look out at the storm and hear the music, and I filled my jam jar again. I drained the pasta and tipped it into the sauce, coating the noodles, and with mouthwatering anticipation, I plated it up. Sitting at the table, I raised my glass to Chet Baker, and Mamma, and to lightning and to bare feet on patio stones and to fresh basil. I dipped my nose down to my plate and let the sweet tangy steam cover my face.

Buon appetito, and sweet dreams.

Spaghetti al Pomodoro

. . . .

SERVES 2 TO 4, DEPENDING ON
HOW MUCH SAUCE YOU LIKE ON YOUR PASTA

As told to me by my wonderful Italian host mother,
Maria Rosaria Carpentieri

From the day I showed up at the Carpentieris's door, I was cared for like a full member of their family. Maybe that's why I turn to this simple but delicious recipe when I want to give myself or someone else a solid dose of nourishment and love. When you are sourcing your ingredients remember that quality matters. Get the best tomatoes and pasta you can, preferably from Italy.

1 can (28 ounces) peeled San Marzano tomatoes
5 tablespoons good-quality olive oil,
     more for drizzling
1/3 white or yellow onion, thinly sliced
Salt
3 fresh basil leaves
1/2 to 1 pound good-quality spaghetti

Turn on some music and clear your workspace so you feel calm and relaxed. Maybe pour yourself something to sip on. It will make a difference in how the food tastes, and anyway, you deserve it.

Open the can of tomatoes and tip them into a medium bowl along with any sauce in the can. Use your hands to break up the tomatoes so that they still have some texture.

Place the olive oil in a large saucepan with a lid over low heat. Add the onion. Cook, uncovered, for about 5 minutes, pushing the onion around with a wooden spoon occasionally, until it is translucent and just a few pieces start to show color.

Tip the tomatoes into the pan with the onions. Add a generous pinch of salt, and the basil. Stir to combine. Cover and let cook on low heat for about 25 minutes. If you like your sauce on the thicker side you can leave the lid off so that more moisture evaporates, though be careful as it might splatter a bit.

While the sauce is cooking, fill a large pot with water, and salt it until it tastes like the sea. Bring the water to a boil. Cook the pasta according to the instructions on the packet. Depending on how many people you are serving or how saucy you like your pasta, you can make anywhere from 1/2 to 1 pound of spaghetti. Half a pound usually works well for 2 people, and 1 pound is good for 4.

Set out bowls and silverware. Refill your drink and hum to yourself.

When the pasta is done, drain it carefully and divide it evenly among the bowls. Taste the sauce and add more salt, if desired. When is tastes right, ladle as much sauce as you like onto each bowl. Finish each serving with a drizzle of olive oil. Sit down and eat. *Buon appetito.*

At the Museum, on a Bright Day

ome save trips to the museum for rainy days.
They wait till it's cold and dreary and let it be the bright
spot on an otherwise gray afternoon. I like to go when it's
bright and sunny, when I'm ready for a break from heat and
the busy noise of the summer.

That day, it had been a week of straight sunshine, long hot days that
I would have begged for in the bitterest part of the winter but that I was
tired of in the summer. I was fussy with the heat and stickiness, and
thinking of the cool quiet of the museum, its open spacious rooms and
wide halls, refreshed me on the spot. Yes, I would make a date with
myself today, and spend all afternoon in the cool hush of the museum
if I liked.

On the front steps of the institute I stopped to look around. The
building took up a full city block, with tall pillars of white sandstone,
splashing fountains that made rainbows on their marble basins, and
patches of tall grasses and sculptures all around. The steps were deep
and accommodating; you could sit, leaning back on your elbows, listening to the fountains; in your own bubble of calm in the middle of
the rushing city, watching the people come and go. Bright banners

hung from the cornice, calling me to see the new exhibits. I found my membership card in my bag and stepped up to the entrance.

It was free to enter, but the year before I'd bought a membership. I guess there were some perks to it, early notice of new events, a discount on tickets for the film festival, but mostly it felt like a small way to vote for a place like this, so that it could keep existing and doing what it was doing when no one was looking. Even if I didn't come for a few months, I'd see the card in my wallet, and I'd feel like I was a part of art and appreciation, like I had a toe dipped into the vast ocean of human creativity, and I liked that.

Stepping into the open space inside, I looked down at the patterns in glossy green-and-white marble built into the floors. I looked up at the startlingly high ceilings, edged with carved molding and sculpted faces. I looked around at the people starting to wander—some, like me, with hands clasped behind their backs (perhaps we were remembering being told on a visit when we were kids to keep our hands to ourselves), and some in small groups moving slowly together from room to room.

I had a friend many years ago who taught me the best way to view art. She said that while it was fine to go to a gallery with a friend, once you were inside there should be no talking. In fact, she said, don't even walk together. Instead set a time to meet for a cup of coffee in the café later and then talk as much as you like. But when you are looking at art you should do it absolutely at your own pace and without the pressure of having to come up with anything clever to say along the way.

I liked this rule. In fact, I took it a bit further and almost always came to places like this alone. How freeing it felt to go as slowly as I liked, to sit and just look at something or nothing at all and to leave whenever I wanted. I shifted my bag across my back, turned toward my favorite gallery, and started my slow walk through the rooms.

I walked through the hall of very ancient art, the oldest the building held. I saw carved pieces of wood and stone shapes worn smooth after years in the wind and rain. I walked through the rooms of old masters, vast landscapes and seascapes, still lifes and dramatic moments in history caught in a single frame. I walked through a courtyard with walls covered in the mural of a modern master of the last century, luckily and carefully preserved, the colors still vibrant. Finally, I came to the portrait gallery. It was darker than the other rooms, and the lights were angled in a way that made you feel, as you stepped up to a painting, that you were having an intimate conversation with the subject, just the two of you.

Some were hundreds of years old, a queen with a dog on her lap, an emperor in a feathered hat with medals draped around his neck. Then a girl at a worktable, her embroidery in hand, a tired look on her face. Some were modern, photorealistic or pixilated: a girl with glowing dark skin and direct confident eyes, a man wrinkled and smudged by the artist with an aura of gray-green around his head. I liked to look at their hands, to consider what they might have been thinking about as their image was taken. Looking around the space at the people in the paintings and those walking around taking them in, I reminded myself, every person is a person—each with their own history and memories and favorite things.

I strolled out into the main hall, my shoes making a soft sound on the marble, and turned toward the new exhibits. I decided I would make my way through them one by one, sit awhile on the bench on the second floor that looked down over the courtyard, then look at the books in the museum shop for a while. Finally, I'd take myself for a sandwich and a cup of tea in the café. I clasped my hands behind my back again and turned down the next hall.

Sweet dreams.

Summer Harvest

We'd gotten here early today, to take advantage of the cool morning air.

The sun was just coming over the trees and the dew was still thick in the grass. We were old hands by now; we knew how to weed, when to water, and mostly when to harvest. We'd had a few missteps along the way. Those potatoes had been tricky, as predicted, but we'd managed to get a small crop of new potatoes and left some in the ground to grow bigger for the fall. I'd been too timid to cut the broccoli, unsure if it was ready, and came one day to find that the beautiful green florets had bloomed into even more beautiful yellow flowers. Oh well. We were learning.

Today we were here to harvest. There would still be much more to come, but the plot was producing so quickly that we'd had to come up with a plan for all we'd grown. We'd brought giant wicker baskets to fill with pounds and pounds of tomatoes. I had a laundry basket lined with an old blanket for the cabbages and cucumbers and zucchini. The runner beans and green beans were mostly finished by now, but we'd left a row of the runners to dry on the vine for winter soups. Those wouldn't be harvested until almost all their leaves had dried and turned brown. When I walked past them, I thought to myself that they would be about ready when the potatoes were. I liked thinking in these terms; instead of Tuesday or Wednesday, instead of one thirty or six o'clock, I kept time based on when the potatoes would be harvested and beans would be cut down and shelled.

We started on the tomato plants, the tangy smell of the vines rubbing off on our hands as we carefully picked the fruit. We had Romas for sauce, huge lopsided heirloom tomatoes for slicing and salads, giant beefsteaks that would go in canning jars that day, and about a million tiny, crisp cherry and grape tomatoes that burst in your mouth with an acidic snap. We took a few that were yet unripe for fried green tomato sandwiches, and some that had fallen heavy and with split skins to the garden floor. We didn't mind their bruises.

We set the full baskets under a tree. The day was getting hotter, and as we stopped for a rest and a cool drink, the family with the allotment next to ours arrived. Their two boys ran to greet us. We were old friends by now. They told us, one talking over the other in a quick galloping rush of words, about summer camp and their new backpacks for school and that their neighbor had a pool (Did we know them? We didn't.) and that later they were going swimming and did we want Popsicles because Mom brought Popsicles. We didn't, but as my friend headed back to the rows to work, I sat for a few minutes at the picnic table under a big maple, and the youngest boy came back, Popsicle in hand, and awkwardly climbed up onto my lap. He swung his feet and contentedly stared into the distance while he ate and dripped his treat onto my dusty work clothes. I rested my chin on his head and hummed a little. When he was done, he handed me the red-stained stick and rushed back to play in the dirt again with his brother.

"Back to work, then," I said, and joined my friend in the rows of zucchini. There were so many zucchini that we were a bit overwhelmed. I'd been grilling it, sautéing it, and baking it into muffins and breads. I'd shredded zucchini on my box grater, sautéed it with olive oil and garlic, and tossed it with pasta. I'd given it to neighbors until they'd refused any more. I remembered an old joke, something my uncle used to say, that if you left your car unlocked in a parking lot this time of year, you'd come back to find it filled with zucchini. We weren't the only growers with an overabundance, but luckily we'd found a food pantry happy to take all that we wanted to give. They'd even set out bins at the entrance to the gardens.

We packed the fruits of our labor into our cars and shook hands, silly and content at the successful completion of the plan we'd made back when the snow was still on the ground. We'd done it. We were farmers now.

From there we headed back to my place to can tomatoes until we dropped. I'd been reading up on canning and had the counters lined with clean new jars, my pressure canner on the stove. There was a lot to do, but before anything else, we needed to eat. I laid out a plate of sliced cucumbers with sea salt sprinkled over them. I'd boiled some of those new potatoes the day before, and cut them into chunks, drizzling them with olive oil and fresh rosemary and salt. That morning, I'd set them out on the counter with a towel draped over the bowl before leaving the house so they'd be room temperature when we were ready to eat. I pulled the towel off the bowl and the smell of the rosemary hit me. Then I turned my attention to the tiny red and orange grape tomatoes and rinsed and halved a mess of them. I drizzled olive oil over them and ripped basil leaves into the bowl. I added salt and a few garlic cloves that I'd peeled and just cut in half. They were there for flavor, not for eating. Then I handed the bowl to my friend and dug out my tomato-salad stirring spoon from the back of the drawer. It was old, from my grandmother's kitchen, and had a long handle, plenty big and deep. I told my friend to stir without stopping for five minutes. She raised an eyebrow but set to work. You can't be too hasty; some things take a long time to cook or combine or ripen or grow, and all you can do is be patient. I turned the broiler on and cut a half dozen thick slices of bread. I laid them out on a sheet pan and drizzled more olive oil, then pushed the slices in.

She stirred; I watched the toasting bread. Bruschetta is meant to be well toasted so that when you top it with the juicy tomato salad it stays crisp. I waited for golden brown and just a little char around the edges and took the bread out.

She dutifully kept to her work with the spoon while I plated up the bread and poured us glasses of tea. "OK," I said, and she brought the bowl over to add to the rest of the feast. The tomatoes had given some of their juice to the oil and the fruit was glossy and fragrant. We piled it onto the warm toasts, picking out the garlic and crunching away with the satisfaction that comes from eating food you've grown yourself. We made our way through the potatoes and cucumbers, and when she sat back with a sigh, I filled her tea glass and broke the last cookie in the jar in half to share.

We looked around the kitchen, taking in the baskets of tomatoes, the rows of jars, and all the work yet to do, but we didn't mind. We'd turn on some music, tidy up the dishes, and start. We'd chat, or work in a comfortable quiet, as we cored and scored the fruit. We'd blanch and shock the tomatoes to take off the skins, then stew them and sterilize the jars. Finally, the jars would go into the canner and, as they came out, we would set them top-down on towels till they cooled. We'd split them up and put them neatly on our pantry shelves for soups and sauces in the winter. We were farmers and now canners as well.

Sweet dreams.

Simple Rosemary Potatoes

. . . . .

MAKES ABOUT 1 QUART

Whenever I make this dish, people don't believe that it's just a few ingredients. I'll recite the recipe and they'll shake their heads and ask, "How can it be so good?" But when you have high-quality ingredients, you don't need anything fancy to make things delicious; in fact, often the flavors are brighter and better when they are allowed to shine by themselves.

> 2.5 pounds Yukon Gold potatoes, peeled and cut into
>   bite-size pieces
> 1/4 cup good-quality olive oil
> Salt
> 2 sprigs fresh rosemary

In a large pot, boil the potatoes for 5 to 6 minutes. When they're done, you want them to hold their shape a bit, not soften as though you are making mashed potatoes with them, so you should feel a tiny bit of resistance when you pierce them with a knife. Drain.

Transfer the potatoes to a large bowl and drizzle with the olive oil. Sprinkle with salt, to taste.

Strip the rosemary leaves from their branches and discard the branches. Roughly chop the leaves. They don't need to be uniform or cut into teeny pieces, you just want to release their oil. Add the rosemary to the bowl and stir to combine.

This dish tastes best at room temperature. Serve it as a side with veggie burgers and salads. The potatoes will keep for 4 days in an airtight container in the fridge.

Back to School

'd been waiting, checking the mail each day for a few weeks, not knowing when it would come.

When it finally showed up—folded around a few envelopes, a flyer for the neighborhood garage sale, and a postcard from a faraway friend—I tucked the other items under one arm and smoothed out the cover. It wasn't a thick catalog, just a couple dozen pages, but it held the promise of something new. I brought everything inside and sat at the kitchen table with a fresh cup of coffee, taking my time to page through the possibilities. I'd finished college long ago but often thought that if I could go back to those days and bring with me the curiosity and focus that had bloomed in me in the years since, I'd enjoy it so much more. I'd have picked my classes with a lot more care, for their subjects rather than their time slots, and studied the things that I'm now so interested in.

A few years ago, I'd taken my nephews for an afternoon of school shopping. They'd already gotten their new clothes and sneakers with their dads, and I'd been allowed to come in at the end for the fun stuff. We'd contemplated all the book bags, notebooks, pencil cases, and boxes of markers. I remembered how important these choices had felt to me when I was their age—how each year's bag or binder had been an attempt to say something about who I thought I might be. Add in the excitement of freshly sharpened pencils and clean blank notebooks and I'd find myself looking forward to a new school year, though I was always sad to see the end of summer. One of my nephews was like me, making slow deliberate choices, asking for advice . . . This one? Or this one? His little brother, silly and carefree, had just tossed things into the cart randomly while I pulled about half of it back out and eventually followed him into the early Halloween section where he stood with a spooky mask and a bag of candy in hand.

When I'd taken them home, we'd sat at their table for a while eating the candy, sharpening their pencils, and setting them up for the first day of school. They'd already gotten their schoolbooks, and I remembered my dad sitting at the table with us when we were their age, carefully covering our books in paper. He'd used brown paper grocery sacks, cutting off the bottoms and opening them at their seams to wrap the paper around the snubbed edges of the much-used books. He'd stack them in front of me as he went, and I'd open my new case of markers and colored pencils and draw out the title and my name, adding in the necessary rainbows and rocket ships. That day with the boys reminded me of how much I'd loved going back to school.

So, I started a new tradition. I decided to learn something new each year when the leaves started to turn. And there I was with my small community-ed catalogue and my coffee and a pencil to make notes in the margins. Last year I'd done a semester of photography and had learned the basics of composition and leading lines and had even developed my own film in the studio darkroom. One year I'd studied genealogy and over the few months of the class had built an extensive family tree. I'd been fascinated by the documents, certificates of birth and death and marriage, and had noticed when looking at my great-grandmother's signature that we'd made our Rs the same way. I'd spent another crisp autumn learning to identify various plants, to forage for stinging nettle, sorrel, and even wild amaranth.

Now, I turned the pages of the catalog and considered what should come next. I folded down the corner of the page on local history; that was tempting, it came with trips to the library and a few local houses and sites. I drew a star beside a course about the basics of space science. I could study white dwarfs, supernovae, neutron stars, and black holes. I was really considering the History of English when I saw one more option—Art Restoration: Step-by-Step.

I carried my coffee into the hall and looked up at a painting that had been handed down over several generations. It showed a woman seated at a table, a book propped open in her hand, and a window behind her looking out on a green landscape. It was full of details, knots and grains in the wood-paneled walls at her back, the soft fold of the fabric in her skirt, a shelf of jars and vases above her head. We'd wondered so many times who the woman was, who had painted her, and if anything could be learned about where she'd come from. But this was all somewhat lost in the layers of dust that had settled on it in the last one hundred and fifty years or so.

I imagined spending the next few months in the broad open art studio of the community center. The woman in the canvas propped on my easel. Me with various brushes and tools, pots of solvent and water and a teacher to help me along the way. I'd clean her canvas and work to reveal the dark smudge in one corner that might possibly be a signature. I'd carefully open the back of her frame and maybe find a label, some scrap of yellowed paper to point me to an archive or a ledger in a library. I strode back to the table, took up my pencil, and circled Art Restoration: Step-by-Step. I might, I thought, solve a mystery.

Sweet dreams.

A Block from Home

I t had been raining since the night before, and there were puddles in the streets.

The sky was gray and low. It was a September afternoon, and it was cool with a breeze that smelled like autumn. I had stopped a block away from my house under the awning of a green-grocer and pulled the collar of my raincoat a bit higher against my cheek. The smell of pears made me turn my head away from the window of the coffee shop on the next corner, where I had been watching a few people sipping from cups and reading newspapers or talking with friends. The pears were small and green but a little soft, with a bruise or two that showed they were ready to be eaten. I asked for two and also for some almonds that the grocer twisted into a piece of brown paper for me. After I tucked my treats into the pocket of my raincoat, I drew my hood back up over my head and crossed the street. I was almost home.

The row of brownstones stood shoulder to shoulder. They were all the same building really, repeated over and over with a few differences in the facades. Some had courtyards, some had gardens and gates, and some had old trees growing up through the cracked

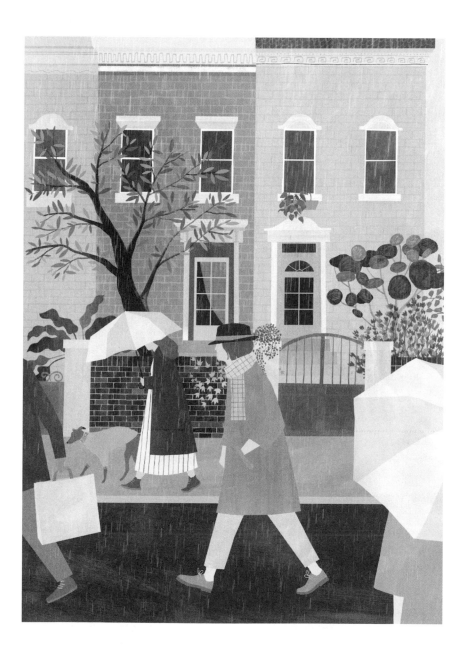

pavements. All of them had wide steps and stoops, though no one was sitting out on them on a day like today.

Mine had a tall wrought iron gate and fence that closed off my slightly overgrown garden from the street. I stopped at the gate and looked for a moment up and down the street: there were a few others making their way through the rain, with heads down or tucked into their umbrellas. I reached into my pocket and pulled out my ring of keys, feeling for the long wrought iron one, heavy and old. My hand always seemed to find it in the dark of my pocket when I was walking. Its weight is reassuring and its long teeth and grapevine handle make it look like it must open a door in a fairy tale. But it doesn't. It opens my gate.

Once through, I heard the gate lock behind me and I hurried past the garden and up to my front door. I'd had enough of the rain. Another key on my ring and I was through with a sigh. I had always enjoyed the feeling of closing the door behind me at the end of the day, knowing I didn't need to leave the house again for the night. Turning back to the door I smiled at the row of locks that ran down the edge of the varnished wood. The door was secure and didn't need them, but I liked to turn them one at a time just the same. I twisted the deadbolt. I slid the chain. I fastened the latch. "Take that, world," I said.

The rain was drumming against the window now, and I looked out at the storm, as it had become a proper storm, before pulling the thick velvet curtain across. I could feel my body becoming heavier with each step. I was just a few minutes away from dropping into a sweet long nap and I knew it. I kicked off my boots and hung my raincoat on the coatrack on my way to the library. Passing through the kitchen with half an idea of having a cup of tea I nearly reached out to press the button on the electric kettle but instantly changed my mind, realizing I'd be asleep before it boiled.

The library had a deep sofa that was long enough to stretch out on and had a couple of throws and pillows. There were reading lamps set here and there but I left them off. The string of fairy lights glowing around the tops of the bookshelves was perfect. I set my pears and almonds on a table beside the sofa and lay down. For a moment, I looked out at the books, with a few snow globes and mementos tucked in. The old clock on the shelf was softly ticking and the rain and thunder were muffled and far away. My eyes were closing. I heard the soft pad of kitty paws, a moment of stillness as she prepared to jump, and then she landed on my knees. I twisted onto my side and she slid into the space behind my legs. I pulled a blanket up over us, laid my face on a soft old pillow, and closed my eyes. We slept.

Sweet dreams.

A SIMPLE RELAXATION TECHNIQUE FOR
WHEN YOU FEEL ANXIOUS AND WORN OUT

. . . . .

I love using this simple method of breathing and counting because it relaxes me almost instantly, and I can do it wherever I am without anyone even noticing. You could try this when you're stuck in traffic, or feeling stressed at work, or when you've had a bad day and you're back at home, wrapped in your favorite hoodie, and need to relax.

Start by breathing naturally and just noticing the way that your breath feels as it moves in and out. You don't need to change anything about it, just pay attention to it. Follow the breath in through your nose, down your throat and into your lungs. Follow it from the lungs back through the throat and nose. When you reach the end of your exhale, count in your head *One, two*. Then, follow the next breath in, and out and again. *One, two*. Do this for a minute or two. In. Out. *One, two*.

When you feel a bit calmer, take a big breath in through your nose and sigh it out through your mouth. Good.

In the Library

hose first few steps into the library always surprise me. I forget, when it's been a while, how quiet and cool it is, how the scent of the books, dusty and sweet, rushes up at you as soon as you open the door, and how keenly inviting the sight of all those books is. Even if I'm just stepping in to return my recent reads, I find I can't help but walk through the stacks for a few minutes and admire the quiet order of the reading rooms. Today I would be there for more than just a few minutes, so I would take my time.

It was my day off, and I'd gotten up early just to make a cup of coffee and crawl back into bed with it. I'd opened the shades in my bedroom and lounged with my cup, looking out at the changing light for a while. I listened to my kitty, purring on the blanket beside me. She was lazily looking out the window too, and every now and then her tail would flick suddenly and then, like a wisp of smoke from a blown-out candle, it would curl and slowly settle back to the bed. I wondered what made that flick happen. What were her kitty thoughts stirred by? I laid a hand on her back and felt the soothing thrum of her purr. I smiled to myself as I made my plans for the day. We were in the first cool days of autumn, leaves just beginning to shift and fall. The nights were getting colder, but by midday the sun warmed the air and it was pleasant to wear a sweater and feel the sun on your back and the cool air on your face. I decided to walk to town and spend some time in the stacks at my library.

I slung a bag with a few necessities across my body and tied my shoes and stepped out to breathe in the midmorning air. I saw a few people walking dogs or bringing in groceries as I made my way through the neighborhood streets and closer to town. It was a little city, really just a few major streets and side alleys, but we had a couple nice cafés, an old cinema with a pretty marquee where they always showed one old movie along with the new ones, a big green park in the center of town, and a really good library.

I got there just a few minutes after they opened, but there were already a few bikes parked at the rack and a steady stream of patrons coming and going, some with children hanging from each hand, others with serious-looking book bags, laptops peeking out, ready to get to work, and some like me, just looking to be close to books and curious to see what they might find. I slid in through the glass front doors and took a moment to look around. I could head straight into the stacks or take the scenic route through the children's section. I picked scenic and took a few minutes to wander past the big storybooks and tiny chairs. I smiled at a dad sitting in the middle of an aisle with his daughter on his lap as they read, and I nodded at the librarians as they re-shelved books and tidied up the desk.

In one of the main rooms, there were neat rows of tables, broad empty workspaces, with identical reading lamps, old chairs, and wastebaskets. I loved the sameness repeating through the space. It made me feel calm and focused. I found a spot for myself, set my bag down, and took a thermos of tea from it and set it out on the desktop. Then I looked around at the rows of books and started to wander the aisles. I let my eyes move over the titles. Like any reader I have my favorites, but I always browsed in unfamiliar sections. That is one of the really exciting things about being surrounded by so many books; when they are all around you, you can just pull one down and start reading, never knowing if you will find the one that opens you up and makes you wonder or laugh or cry or just live differently thereafter.

I'd planned to get only a book or two, but after an hour of browsing and sampling I had five. I was sitting for a few minutes back at the neat desks, sipping tea and skimming pages, deciding which one I would start first, when my stomach gave a low warning rumble. I thought about staying put a bit longer, but since one of the only things more enjoyable than reading a new book is reading a new book while you eat a sandwich, I decided to check out my armful of fresh picks and go.

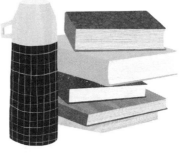

In the park, there was a kiosk that sold ice cream and coffee and sandwiches and cold drinks. I lined up with some office workers on their break and waited my turn to order "the one with lots of pickles on it, please." They wrapped it up in brown paper for me, gave me an apple as well, and sent me on my way. I settled onto a bench in a quiet corner of the park, unwrapped my sandwich, and noticed the cool autumn air around me. It was the perfect day for a new book. I'd always thought that each season had its own best sort of leisurely pursuit. Winter was for movies. Spring was for poetry. Summer was for music. And autumn, autumn was for books.

I'd checked out a book about the cosmos and concepts that I'd always wanted to understand but never had, a mystery set in an English country house, a memoir, a novel that I'd picked up just because I'd liked the cover, and a book about what might have happened if lots of things in Earth's history had gone just a bit differently. I thumbed through the book with the pretty cover; it had, unexpectedly, beautiful illustrations and engravings throughout. I read a bit, then shifted to the memoir for a moment, noticing where a few pages had been folded over by a previous reader. I knew I was going to go straight for the country house mystery (and hope that the butler hadn't done it), but I pretended for a few more minutes that I might finally read about the multiverse and string theory. Then, brushing the crumbs off my lap, I opened my new book and started to read.

Sweet dreams.

That is one of the really
exciting things about being
surrounded by so many
books; when they are all
around you, you can just
pull one down and start
reading, never knowing if
you will find the one that
opens you up and makes
you wonder or laugh or
cry or just live differently
thereafter.

At the Farmers Market,
on a Fall Morning

I t used to be that Saturday mornings were for sleeping till noon . . . and sometimes for piecing together the night before from blurry memories.

But I guess I've grown up a bit because now I look forward to being up early and having the whole day laid out in front of me to plan and enjoy.

That morning, I was sitting on the back porch, wrapped in a blanket, with a cup of tea in my hands, enjoying its fragrant steam rising against my cheek in the chill. I'd been watching a squirrel gathering acorns and hiding them away in her secret spots in the yard. I guessed we were making the same plans this morning, gathering the harvest and thinking ahead to winter, as that day I was heading to the farmers market to fill my bags with all the good things that come with the end of the summer and peak of the autumn.

I set my teacup in the sink and stepped out into the garage. I nearly rode my bike instead and left the car at home, but I knew myself too well. I would surely buy more than I could ever carry on my bike, especially now that pumpkins and squashes were filling up the market stalls. The market was busy by the time I arrived, and I circled for a few minutes looking for a place to park. I went all the way to the back of the lot and slipped my car into a spot and stepped out into the crisp morning. Just beyond the last row of cars stood a circle of tall trees, their leaves starting to turn and fall in the morning breeze; at their feet was an old tilting bench and the bank of a creek running swiftly by. I took a minute, with my market bags tucked under my arm, to squat down on a flat rock by the water and watch it flow past. The water was cool and I let my fingers trail through it and smelled the mixture of the fresh water with the spicy morning air. I took a few deep breaths, then turned back to the market and followed the stream of people and kids and dogs to the overflowing stalls.

I knew from experience that the best strategy was to walk the length of the market, just looking first, not buying till I knew what was available and where the best bits were, but I'm not good at waiting, especially when surrounded by so much abundance. I've made peace with that, and now I just accept that I'll buy too much and struggle to get it back to the car.

Mums were stacked along the walkway and up on old milk crates, some with their buds fully open and others still tucked in, their blossoming a ways off yet. Behind them, on broad wooden benches, were jars of sunflowers and pots of zinnias and pansies, decorative cabbages and purple kale. I paid for a few things and arranged to pick them up on the way out, then headed over to the banks of vegetables and stacks of pumpkins. There were still tomatoes coming in, and I bought some for canning, along with lumpy yams and a sugar pumpkin to roast and puree into a soup. I bought a whole branch of brussels sprouts and butternut squash and chard with bright yellow stems.

My bags were heavy on my shoulders, but I persisted and made my way past the open-air stalls into the enclosed market with the bustling crowd. There, I bought a jar of pumpkin butter, great stuff that I had bought before and could be used to turn a humble piece of toast into something like pumpkin pie for breakfast. Sign me up. At the far end of the market was a bakery whose sweet smells permeated clear to the parking lot. The line for their goods was a few patrons deep and I used my time waiting to take in the yeasty hot smell of fresh bread and pastries and cookies. I had a distinct memory of being a child, maybe five or six at the time, and standing in the same spot, holding my mother's hand as she bought a dozen chocolate-chip cookies in a white paper bag. Even all these years later, there were stacks of the same bags held in place against the breeze with a rock beside the register. As the baker turned her expectant face to me and took my order, she used a piece of waxed paper to slip a loaf of pecan cinnamon bread into one. I paid the baker, shifted the bags onto my shoulders, and stepped back out into the brisk open air.

As predicted, it took two trips to get everything buckled into the car. As I was tucking in the stems of my mums and pansies and closing the hatch door, I smelled coffee and hot cider, and I noticed a squat shiny cart parked at the far end of the lot. I still had a few dollars left, so I bought myself a coffee and sat at a picnic table, people watching while I drank it. Someone was playing a guitar nearby, a girl was telling a friend a story that had them both giggling until one was wiping her eyes, head thrown back in a roar of laughter. A few feet away an older couple held hands and walked in slow, patient steps past the vegetable vendors. The chill of the day was working its way up into my legs, so I stood up and, taking the last few sips of my coffee, headed back to the car to see what the rest of my Saturday would become.

Sweet dreams.

PEOPLE WATCHING AS MEDITATION

. · . · .

This meditation is a nice way to feel centered when you're somewhere busy.

Find someplace out of the way where you can sit without being bumped into. Put both feet flat on the floor and sit in a way that is comfortable but with an upright spine.

Focus your eyes on something that isn't moving, and isn't a person, and pay attention to the sensations in your own body. Notice the rhythm of your breath and the way your clothes feel against your skin. After a few moments like this, let your eyes start to move slowly over the people around you. Without forming any opinions about the people you see, just take in the details of what they are doing, how they are moving, the color of their hair or the shape of their eyes. Curiously gather details as if you were an artist preparing to paint the scene in front of you.

Periodically check back in with the feelings inside your own body, then look at the world around you again. Remember that meditation is just paying attention in a calm way, and you can do it when you're sitting, walking, eating, or in the middle of a crowd.

Breathe in. Breathe out. Good.

Rosemary, for Remembrance

I was out in my vegetable garden.

By now, it had mostly been tilled down back into the earth after the last ears of corn were eaten. I wanted to harvest the last few bits that the garden could give us before the hard frost set in.

I started with my section of soft-skinned gourds, called *Cucurbita*. They grew with long hooked necks and knobbly, shiny skin. They were green and gold, or a bright sunrise orange-red, and most were small enough to be carried in one hand. I cut them from the vine and heaped them into wooden baskets. They'd decorate my table, sit in wreaths of bright red maple leaves on my porch, and the extras would be set out at the edge of the woods for any passing animal in search of a nibble.

I moved to my hard-skinned gourds, called *Lagenaria*. These were a tan, sandy brown and quite large—in fact, some had grown almost as big as my pumpkins. I harvested them one at time, leaving a few inches of vine on the stem and carrying each one to the spigot at the edge of the barn. I washed each gourd carefully in the cold water of the tap, and when I was done, I laid them out on an old patched quilt in the autumn sunlight to dry.

The gourds would cure over the winter and their insides would slowly dry till they were as light as paper. I had a spot in the barn, warm enough that they wouldn't freeze in the depth of the winter but dry, and where the air could move around them. I'd set them out in a long row on a shelf, with a bit of space between them, giving them a turn every couple of months. In the spring, when they finally rattled when shook, their seeds dancing around inside the hard skin, I'd carefully cut into them to make an open space to fill with birdseed and a slot to thread a bit of rope. I'd hang them out to feed the black-capped chickadees, the cerulean warblers, and the yellow-breasted chats. I might paint some in shades of sky blue or shiny black and give them to friends and neighbors.

After the gourds, I spent some time cutting pumpkins from their vines and placing them in a row at the end of the long gravel drive. We had more than we could use or eat, so I set out a hand-stenciled sign asking a few dollars per pumpkin and left an old coffee can to collect my earnings on top of the mailbox.

Soon enough, I heard the crunch of tires on the drive and looked up to see a couple and a little boy inspecting the pumpkins. The boy squatted down to run his tiny hands over the smooth bright orange skin and the prickly green stem. It's a big decision to a little one . . . Which pumpkin is the right one? After a minute he picked one and though it took him a few tries he got his arms around it and shuffled it back to their car. I saw his mom push a few bills into the coffee can, and she raised an arm to wave at me in the garden. I waved back and moved on to my herb garden.

I'd already cut the last of the parsley, oregano, and basil in September, but there was still plenty of sage and sorrel and thyme. The thyme in particular smelled so good as it warmed in the sun that I rubbed it between my palms and then cupped them in front of my face. I closed my eyes and pulled in several slow breaths. Rudyard Kipling wrote that thyme smelled like dawn in paradise.

Thinking of the poetry of plants and herbs, I reached out to prune the last branches of rosemary. "There's rosemary, that's for remembrance. Pray you, love, remember. And there's pansies, that's for thoughts." I said it aloud, though I was no Ophelia. I wasn't brokenhearted or lost; instead, when I was in my garden I was found.

I stood a moment, pressing down through the toes of my shoes into the garden. Maybe I was trying to connect my body directly into the earth to say thank you, to say "I am noticing how much you give and I am grateful." I remembered a moment years earlier when I'd told a friend that I felt a strong need to be out in nature. He'd said with kindness in his voice "You are nature." Of course, he was right, and I'd carried that remembrance with me during times I couldn't be in the open fresh air or touch the soil or walk in the thick groves of trees.

I cut bunches of sage for our Thanksgiving dinner and stems of catnip for the felines in the family. I piled a few inches of pine needles 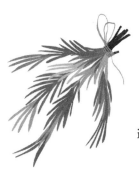 over the pruned stems of the rosemary to protect her from the frost and snow that would come, and I tucked a branch into the front pocket of my old flannel shirt so that the perfume would follow me all day. Rosemary was for remembrance and I was remembering my place in the nature of things.

Sweet dreams.

CURING A GOURD

· · · · ·

Start with a hard-skinned gourd, the larger tan type. Wash it with soap and water and let air dry.

Rub the skin of the gourd with rubbing alcohol to ensure further drying.

Set your gourd in a well-ventilated space out of direct sunlight. Let rest for 6 months, turning it once a week or so to ensure it dries evenly. If it becomes moldy or begins to rot, discard and begin again with a new one. When the gourd is fully cured, it will be light, and will rattle when you shake it.

Cured gourds make pretty additions to indoor or outdoor decorations. They are strong and long lasting, but very light. You can cut into them to make a bird feeder, paint them with oil-based or acrylic paint, or set them out just as they are on your table or front porch.

Canceled Plans

t had seemed like a good idea at the time.

Doesn't it always? Friday night, a movie we both wanted to see and a restaurant we both liked, and the next day off to sleep in if we stayed out a little too late.

But it had been a long day already. I'd been rushing and racing since I'd left the house that morning. I'd forgotten my lunch at home and had gotten by with an apple and some crackers I'd found in my desk. Still, I was hungry. I was also tired—I longed to be in my softest clothes and to be alone and do whatever I pleased. It had started raining on my way home, a cold rain that pushed under my collar and chilled my hands. The thought of fixing myself up and heading right back out into the gloomy weather was a miserable one.

Luckily, the friend I had plans with was a good one, one who had sworn a promise with me years ago: we'd both pledged to always be honest about what we could or couldn't do, what we wanted and didn't want. That way we knew that when we asked for a favor or to share an adventure and the other said yes, they did it with their whole heart and not out of obligation. And if they said no, then it meant that the other person was just taking care of themselves and that felt good too. So I didn't debate long. I picked up my phone and saw that she and I, as had happened so often before, were already in sync. She'd sent a message, just one word.

Ummm . . .

I laughed with my phone in my hand and sent back:

You too?

I'm already in my jammies.

Good. Stay that way. We'll go another day. XO

XO

"Yes!" I called out, pumping one fist into the air. I took a deep breath and sighed it out. I hadn't realized I'd been hunching my shoulders and clenching my jaw until I felt everything relax. Now that I knew I was staying in, I took my time. I peeled off my wet coat and hung it by the door, then went to my bedroom and pulled out my favorite pajamas, a pair of thick socks, and an old soft cardigan. Since I was still chilled from the rain, I took those cozy clothes to the dryer and pushed them in. I set it to run for ten minutes and in the meantime drifted through the house lighting candles and turning on music. I looked through the fridge and leafed through the drawer of takeout menus and considered what I was hungry for. I thought about ordering a pizza or some spicy Thai vegetables and noodles, but I felt a bit bad making the delivery person come out on this rainy, chilly night. I heard the dryer ding and excitedly raced over to it. It's funny what becomes exciting as we get older. I'd been worn out and exhausted when I got home. Now I was energized and animated, eagerly looking forward to doing next to nothing all on my own.

The clothes were wonderfully hot as I took them from the dryer and changed into them before they could lose any warmth. I pulled the thick socks onto my feet and felt my toes finally warming up. I wrapped the cardigan over my pajamas and let myself flop back onto my bed. It just felt so good to be home; I wondered if I would have enjoyed it this much if I'd never intended to go out. Something about comparing one against the other made this option much sweeter. I found my phone and sent another message to my friend.

"Let's cancel plans again next weekend."

She sent back, "Can't wait. There's a concert downtown."

"I'm so excited to not go to it."

I liked knowing we were both cozily tucked into our homes, she relaxed and happy across town and me here, finally warming up in mine. It's the best version of friendship: when someone else's happiness makes you happy even though you aren't there to see it.

Back in the kitchen, I went through the fridge again and came away with a package of cremini mushrooms and some fresh parsley. In the pantry I found broth and arborio rice and a bottle of wine. Risotto was the perfect meal on a night like tonight. It was hearty and filling and comforting and warm, as well as downright delicious. I set a wide pan on the stove and diced onions and cooked them slowly in olive oil. In a separate pan I started warming the broth. I uncorked the wine, pouring some for me and keeping the bottle handy to deglaze the pan.

When my onions began to smell heavenly and were just a bit rosy,

I added the rice to the pan and stirred it through for a minute or so. The outer hull of the grains became translucent with a pearly heart visible beneath. I started to slowly ladle hot broth into the rice, one spoonful at a time, stirring and letting the broth absorb before adding more. It was like a meditation, drawing my wooden spoon through the pan and watching the creamy sauce form as the rice gave up its starch and softened. Another ladle, more stirring. I let the savory steam warm my face and neck as I stood over the pans.

I stepped away, to chop parsley to sprinkle on top and quarter the mushrooms, which I sautéed separately, with a bit of the wine, to add right at the end. Turning off the heat, I tipped the mushrooms into the rice, then stirred it through with generous pinches of salt and pepper.

Finally, I ladled it up into a bowl. My stomach was growling in anticipation as I carried dinner to the coffee table. Yes. I was going to eat wrapped in a blanket on the couch, watching a movie. I was a grown-up and nobody could stop me.

"Harrumph," I said to no one.

I set myself up, feet propped up, bowl in my lap, wineglass in my hand, and turned on the TV. I'd been saving a movie for a night just like this. I'd meant to see it in the theater. The memory made me laugh. I'd probably made plans with my friend to go and we had canceled. It was a whodunit with an ensemble cast full of favorite actors, set a hundred years ago with beautiful sets and locations. A long time ago, I'd read the book it was taken from but had forgotten who the killer was, so I was ready to play detective as I watched. The rain beat against the windows behind me. I took a slow sip from my glass and pressed play.

Sweet dreams.

INSTRUCTIONS FOR FEELING
BETTER AFTER A BAD DAY

· · · · ·

Some days are not so great. Some days are just bad. So, when you get home at the end of one of those days, stand in the kitchen for a bit and make a big cup of hot chocolate. You can add a handful of chocolate chips and stir them in to make it a bit nicer. Or you can make a cup of tea, milky and sweet with a good pour of whiskey in it. You can say to yourself while you're adding the whiskey, "Practically medicinal." But you don't need to. You can have it just because you want it.

Then, walk around the house checking the locks, and when you turn the last one, say to the world, "Stay out there." Then, go to your bedroom, set your cocoa by the bed, and turn on just one small lamp. Find the softest pajamas you own, the ones that have been washed a hundred times and are so soft and cool and thin that just slipping them over your legs make you sigh in relief. Then a big soft hoodie. Zip it up and pull the hood over your head. Socks might help.

Now get back to bed. If there is a person there, you can crawl into their lap and let them rub your head while you close your eyes. If there is a dog or a kitty, they will curl up with you and warm you with their quick beating hearts. If you are alone, relax knowing that you can show just exactly how you feel and don't need to explain it to anyone. If the phone rings, you don't have to answer it. If there are messages and things you didn't finish today, you can leave them till tomorrow. That's enough for today.

Sip your chocolate. Turn the light off. Pull the blanket over your shoulder. Take your mind somewhere soft and simple. Breathe in . . . and out. Breathe in . . . and out.

At the Mill, with Pumpkins and Cider

T hrough the heat of the summer, I'd been waiting.

And now, it was here. The cool crisp autumn had arrived and with it that feeling of energy and refreshment that replaces the drowsy languor of the summer. The afternoon light was golden in the way that only ever happens in the fall, the air smelled sweet and spicy, and the leaves were turning, making a new landscape for each passing day. Years ago, I had said to a friend that my eyes were so hungry for the colors of the leaves that I felt like I couldn't look hard enough. She'd smiled and said, "Soften your focus." It was good advice; the moments I looked forward to were best enjoyed with patience and calm attention.

That morning, looking out at the changing colors and feeling the cool air on my face, I stood still for a bit and softened my focus. I even closed my eyes and just listened to the sound of wind moving through drying leaves, a different sound from the breeze in the summer, when the leaves are fresh and still green, but one that could have easily been missed if I hadn't stood so still or listened so long.

Afterward, we'd spent the morning raking leaves and putting away pots and coiling up hoses into the dark corner of the garage. There were mums, purple and rust red, on the porch, but as we stood hands on hips to admire them, we agreed something was missing.

"I guess we need some pumpkins," I said.

"I guess so." A smile, bright eyes.

"And some cider?"

"Obviously."

We pulled on the sweaters that we'd shrugged off in the heat of yard work and jumped in the car. We headed out, main roads to side roads to dirt roads, an old song on the radio that I knew half the words to, our fingers interlaced on the armrest. Rows and rows of knobbly squat apple trees, low and heavy with fruit, were sliding past the windows, and we finally pulled the car into a grassy rutted lot in front of the mill. In tall wooden bins along the front of the barn and shop were apples, so many apples, the ones you wait for all year because they taste and smell so much better than the ones at the store. There were also piles of pumpkins, rows of pumpkins, fields of pumpkins, along with folks walking through, carefully deliberating, then claiming, "This one's mine."

Inside were shelves of preserves, cold cases full of fresh cider, and trays of hot donuts. Some were bare, just crisp and plain, others rolled in sugar or dipped in icing. Through one wall of the little shop was an old arched doorway into the pressing room where you could watch the cider being made. We stopped a moment there and watched a little boy watch the press come down. Why is it so fascinating to watch how things are made?

I thought back to the grainy videos watched on rainy half days in elementary school, remembered being mesmerized by a short of how crayons were made: Hundreds of naked blue crayons, skimming down a conveyor belt headed for their wrapping and then tucked neatly into boxes, the boxes into crates, the crates onto trucks. The memory made me smile at the boy, who stood mesmerized with a finger pressed in concentration to his chin while his father squatted down behind him and pointed out the mechanism that was making his cup of cider. He has so many autumns ahead of him.

Back outside we headed to the pumpkin fields, kicking through fallen leaves and looking out past the edge of the orchard to the rolling land, smoothed in some places after the harvest, and crowded with groves of trees and edged by a quick moving creek in others. We found a batch of tall pumpkins with flattish bottoms and green gnarled stems that looked like they came from a fairy tale. We scooped them up along with some tiny round pumpkins, bright orange and just asking to have a face carved onto them, and carried the whole lot back in to have them weighed on an old rusty scale by the register (forty cents a pound). Along with a brown paper bag of apples and a quart of cold cider, we had everything we'd come for and more.

Back at home, we set out our pumpkins on the stoop and sat down beside them to enjoy the last of both the cider and the evening light. Soon we would put away the rakes and tidy the last pots and yard bags. Soon we would head in and light some candles and start to fix dinner. But just now, just for a few more minutes, we sat and let the cool air chill our necks and noses. Just now we listened for the evening sounds of birds and chipmunks settling into bed and looked out at the changing colors of the night sky. Just now we softened our focus and forgot to be busy.

Sweet dreams.

Secret Admirer

I was fishing around for my keys, and when I pulled them out a tiny scrap of paper came with them.

It caught in the wind for a moment and I quickly reached up to snatch it back. I figured it was a gum wrapper or a movie stub, but when I unfolded it I found a small handwritten note:

You're lovely.

Beside the words was a little sketch of a heart struck through with an arrow. I stood stock-still and smiling, and even though a cool wind was pushing into the folds of my coat, I suddenly felt warm all over.

I slipped my key into the lock and opened my front door, then closed the door behind me and read the note again. Although, it was just two words, so I guess reading wasn't really what I was doing. Instead, I was letting the feeling of being thought of fondly by someone somewhere wash through me. It felt like giddiness and warmth and an excited hollowness in my stomach. I hung my coat on the rack by the door and thought a moment about where and when this note might have found its way into my pocket.

you're lovely 💛

I'd started the day at the bakery and had draped my coat over the back of a chair as I sat and sipped on a coffee. I'd been looking through my planner, making notes and plans for the week. Would I have noticed if someone had passed beside me for a moment to drop the note into my pocket? Probably not. I'd sat for some time and had gotten up for a second cup and a pastry filled with jam. The pastry was crisp and flaky and delicious, and I'd savored it slowly; at that point there could have been an earthquake and I wouldn't have noticed.

From there I'd walked to the library. But no, I'd gone through the park first, where they were setting up booths for an artists market. I stopped to help a few people whose tent flap had come loose and was rippling in the wind. We wrestled it back to its fastenings, and I'd even helped them roll a few pumpkins into place in front of their booth. They had baskets of handmade crafts for fall decorating, and I looked through them for a few minutes. There were wreaths of deep orange and red oak leaves and some spooky bats made with wire and nylon to hang from your front porch. They had skulls and spiders crafted from origami paper and a bag of Honeycrisp apples. They tossed me an apple to thank me for my help, and I slipped it into my bag for later. I didn't think the note could have been

passed to me then—the makers had all been busy unpacking and setting up.

I carried the note to my sofa beside the big bay window that looked
out over the street. The wind was still blowing and the air was swirling with the tiny pale-yellow locust leaves from the trees that lined the
curbs. Their leaves were so small and light that they floated in each
time I opened the front door. I thought of them spinning and drifting
on the wind and wondered if this little note had done the same thing.
Maybe it had already passed from admirer to admired and from there
floated accidentally into my pocket.

But it wasn't creased, and the edges weren't worn. It had been
folded and unfolded only once by the hands who wrote it and then by
my own. I looked with a keen eye at the handwriting and the heart but
couldn't see anything I recognized.

I thought back to where I'd gone from the park. The library had
been my next stop. I'd meant to just push the books I was returning
through the slot in the door and be off to my next errand but I'd gotten
a bit cold, and when I looked through the window at the people browsing shelves and the big overstuffed couches in the reading room, I'd
been pulled right in. I walked past the reference desk and went to the
wall of magazines and newspapers. I loved this part of the library; I
couldn't subscribe to all the magazines I wanted to read each month but
the library could and it meant I got to read articles and look at glossy
pictures and thumb through pages to my heart's content. I plucked a few
from the wall, one about archaeology, which promised a look inside a
recently discovered tomb, one with stories and pictures about new ideas
in architecture, and one with hearty recipes for cold weather. There was

a row of armchairs by the sofas, and though some were taken up with a few other readers I found a spot to stretch out and flip through pages, reading and looking at pictures. I added a few things to my grocery list and eventually set the magazines back in their place. Had anyone bumped into me, slyly slipping me this note? It was possible.

From the library I'd gone to buy a birthday card at the stationery shop. I'd written my message inside with a borrowed pen at their sales desk and taken it straight to the post office to buy a stamp and send it on its way. I went to the market to buy a few things for dinner and stopped to look at a pair of shoes in a store window.

I'd been many places, passed crowds of people.

I realized that as I was retracing my steps, thinking back through the day, I was looking for one specific face to show up in the crowd. The face of a someone who I was secretly hoping had written and slipped me this note. It had been a while since I was in school, but it seemed I wasn't too old to have a crush, to be smitten, and to enjoy just thinking about someone.

Romance is often at its best when it's still in the theoretical stage, so I decided to stop searching my memory and to just enjoy the possibility that the person whom I admired also admired me back. That they had seen me on the street today and hadn't been able to help themselves from scratching out this heart and these words and, with their pulse rising, had dropped their feelings into my coat pocket.

I'd find a special place to keep my note and perhaps one day could confirm my hopeful suspicions.

Sweet dreams.

Halloween, in an Old House

As I looked through my closet a few hours before the trick-or-treating was likely to begin, I remembered traveling through Europe years ago.

I was stepping down onto a train platform and was stopped in my tracks by the thought that in that moment I could be anybody. None of the people spilling past me knew anything about me. I could reinvent myself if I liked, claim a different name, speak with an accent, be brave about things I hadn't been brave about before, or just try on a different kind of life. Doesn't Halloween have the same appeal? It's the chance to try on something different—a mask, a costume— a day when we all allow each other a bit of strangeness.

I pushed through the hangers and found a black overcoat that could be made to look a bit like a witch's robe. I clucked my tongue: not a witch again. Past that I found an old dress, long and scarlet, cut a bit close with a high waist. All right, all right, I'd had a *Pride and Prejudice* phase; we were all young once. On a hook beside the dress was a crown, silly, golden, and bedazzled, something I'd been given to wear at a bachelorette night out. I looked at the crown and the dark red dress and slipped a necklace off a hook, a costume piece with a big red heart hanging from it.

"Queen of Hearts?"

"Bump," said the attic.

"Thank you for your opinion." I smiled up at the ceiling above.

The attic didn't usually have much to say. Once, maybe twice a day there was a soft inconspicuous bump, as if someone had just set their coffee mug down a bit hard on a table or closed a book for the night. In fact, it was usually in the evening: ten minutes or so before bedtime, I'd hear that muffled thump and I'd set down my book and call out "Me too then; lights out, shall we? Sleep tight." All old houses are likely to have strange sounds and flickering lights, but honestly that bump had always felt like a friendly wave from a neighbor that you know by sight but not by name. We nodded at each other, then moved on with our days and besides, everyone has to live somewhere.

Queen of Hearts it was then, that was decided. I took the dress out to the landing where a wide window looked down to the street. I opened it and let the cool spicy Halloween air in. I hung the dress from the window sash and leaned out a moment, elbows on the sill, to watch the street. Neighbors were setting out pumpkins on stoops, children were stepping off the bus, kicking through and falling into piles of leaves, already dressed in their costumes. I remembered that giddy thrill of being allowed to wear my costume to school—a whole day lost to parties and parades and candy. The excitement of children is completely untempered, undiluted, and even at this distance it was contagious. I drummed my fingers on the sill, then spun on my heel and headed down into the kitchen.

I'd done the pumpkin carving earlier, an old monster movie playing in the background while I scooped out the seeds and cut silly faces in. The seeds were roasting in the oven now and by the smell they were just about done. I'd coated them with olive oil and sea salt and black pepper, and when I popped a few into my mouth they sizzled on my tongue deliciously. I spooned them into a bowl for snacking on while I handed out treats. I bustled around the house, lighting candles and getting my giant treat bowl ready.

Finally, I took out my pumpkins and set them up on my front steps. I amused myself for a while setting them up in different scenarios, this pumpkin is in love with that one and this one's jealous . . . I was having a bit too much fun for a grown-up alone on her porch on Halloween, but I looked around and didn't see anyone watching, so I carried on for a bit.

The light was changing; at this time of year, sunset happens in just a few minutes, and dusk goes to darkness quickly. I lit the candles in the jack-o'-lanterns and rushed back upstairs to get into my dress and crown. The landing was chilly now, and I closed the window and pulled my dress down from its spot. As I turned to head back to my room, I stopped short.

The attic stairs had dropped down from the ceiling and were resting on the landing floor. They were those old sort of retractable steps you pulled a cord from the ceiling to release, but I hadn't pulled the cord. I took a deep breath.

"Very well," I said calmly, "I suppose if there is one night of the year when you are allowed to act up a bit, it's Halloween night." I took the ensuing silence for agreement.

I edged around the steps and into my room, closing the door behind me as I got into my dress. There was a lingering chill in my body, that was certain, but I remembered the excitement of the kids gearing up for their neighborhood prowl and how it had gotten into my system a bit ago, and I thought that it must be even more contagious than I'd imagined.

I settled my crown onto my head and looped the silly heart necklace around my throat, slipped my feet into some old red velvet slippers, and heard the first call of "Trick-or-treat!" from the front door.

"We'd better get down there," I called out.

"Bump," said the attic.

Sweet dreams.

Crispy Roasted Pumpkin Seeds

. . . . .

MAKES 1 CUP

You are never too old to carve a pumpkin or to enjoy a delicious treat like these. They are particularly nice on Halloween night, when you've been sneaking candy from the trick-or-treat bowl and need something salty to cut through the sugar.

1 cup raw pumpkin seeds, separated as much as possible
    from the pumpkin flesh
1 tablespoon extra virgin olive oil or melted coconut oil
Salt, to taste
1/2 teaspoon ground cumin (optional)
Pinch of cayenne pepper (optional)

Preheat the oven to 325°F. Line a large plate with a paper towel. Line a baking sheet with parchment paper.

Remove as much pumpkin flesh as possible from the pumpkin seeds. Wash the pumpkin seeds and let dry on the paper-towel–lined plate. Pat dry with an additional paper towel, if necessary.

In a medium bowl, combine the pumpkin seeds, oil, salt, and spices, if using. Toss well, until all the seeds are evenly coated.

Spread the seed mixture onto the baking sheet. Use a spoon to arrange the seeds in a single layer.

Bake for 20 to 30 minutes, until golden brown and crispy. Larger seeds take longer to bake, smaller seeds take less time.

Enjoy! The roasted seeds can be kept in a sealed glass jar at room temperature for up to a week.

Tools on the Workbench

y sister is a maker, a maker of all sorts of things.

Our father had been the same, and when we were young, they'd spent a lot of time in our garage on rainy spring afternoons or in the heat of summer with the garage door open and fresh air coming in as they tinkered away.

My father could often be found turning a piece of wood on the lathe, shaping it with sharp, attentively held tools as it went around. He loved creating tiny details in the pieces he made, details that might go unseen by most but were cherished by the few who took time to really look. When I was very young, he'd made me a small writing desk that included a handful of tiny and beautiful features that must have taken him ages to create: a lid that, when raised, slid cleanly into a pocket hidden in the top of the desk and, when lowered, could be locked by a tiny wrought iron key that clipped onto my charm bracelet. A drawer on one side, with a hidden catch that opened a panel carved with my initials. It was pretty much the best gift I'd ever received. In a world where so much seems to be made just to be thrown away, the things he created were real treasures.

While my father was carving and sanding and staining, my sister was tinkering and taking things apart. She collected old clocks and other bits of unwanted and broken machinery from neighbors and methodically disassembled them on her own small workbench. She'd patiently back screws out of their holes and lift out the tiny wheels and cogs of a thing's inner workings, running her hands over the pieces to see where some tooth or spoke was broken or twisted. She mended and reassembled, and soon the piece would be ticking or whirring away on her bench. Our dad would look over and give her a proud smile and they'd each turn to the next project.

I would flit in and out as they worked, trying to keep my hands in my pockets and not interrupt their concentration. While they were lovers of details, I preferred a grander scope and struggled to keep my focus on one project or place. They'd patiently explain what they were working on when I asked but weren't surprised when, a moment later, I was climbing onto my bike for long ride or sketching the lines of the sunset into the sawdust on the floor.

Years later I am still scattering my attention in lots of directions, and my sister is still a maker. Recently, I called her when I'd found something at a flea market that I thought was worthy of her workshop. I'd been out driving on a crisp autumn day taking in the colors of the turning leaves when I'd seen a sign for an outdoor market. On a whim, I'd pulled over and walked into the maze of booths and stalls. There were racks of vintage varsity jackets, with well-worn patches and names embroidered in gold thread. There were old milk crates filled with records from the fifties and sixties.

I found an old tin cake carrier that was only slightly banged up and had a slot on the bottom to slip a knife into. Just the thing for taking a cake on a picnic, a thing which I would almost certainly never do but it was so charming and only a few bucks so I added it to my collection.

Before I left, I found a small wooden music box, inlaid with crumbling velvet, which tried half-heartedly to spring to life when I opened it. Inside was a tiny carved girl on ice skates endeavoring to spin along the track cut into the box's interior, around a snow-covered pine tree and a stag standing proudly in a drift. I tried the key at its back but it felt already as if it had been too tightly wound, and afraid I would further break it, I carefully closed the lid, paid a few dollars for it, and carried it back to the car.

My sister invited me straight to her workshop, promising to put on a pot of coffee in the meantime. Soon we were standing there, hot cups in our hands, with the little box in front of us. Where my father had been a bit casual about his tools, my sister was fastidious. The walls were lined in pegboards with tools hanging in organized, graduated rows. It was immensely satisfying to see each thing in its place, a large screwdriver with a slightly smaller one hanging beside it and an even smaller one beside that. There were neat bins of reclaimed parts and lengths of wood, metal drawers with sheets of sandpaper organized by their grit, and tiny plastic trays with every imaginable length and shape of fastener. There were shelves of old manuals with strands of twine stuck in to mark a page and bins of magazines dating back to my father's time. The place had the good clean smell of wood shavings and was quiet except for the sound of a couple of ticking clocks my sister had rebuilt and proudly hung from the walls.

She slipped a wide carpenter's pencil behind her ear and took out a box of very small tools from a drawer. She tilted a gooseneck lamp toward her work and started to slowly take the music box apart. As she worked, I drifted around the room, sipping coffee and watching leaves fall outside. I paged through a magazine for hobbyists, and when one of the clocks struck the hour, I watched as a small carved door opened in its face and a tiny bird popped out to sing along with the chime. At the same time a wooden figure at its base lifted a minuscule pair of binoculars to its painted eyes to spy the bird. I chuckled at its cleverness. From her bench my sister let out a satisfied sigh, and I turned to watch her slowly wind the key in the back of the music box. I joined her at the bench and we listened to the sweet tinny sound of the tune that was being heard for the first time in decades and watched the skater as she spun and slid around her track.

Not everything that has stopped working has to be thrown away. With a bit of patience and effort, in fact, nearly everything could be repaired and set to making music again.

Sweet dreams.

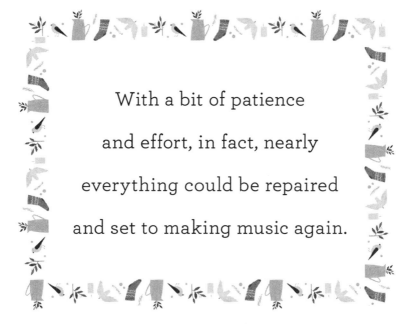

With a bit of patience
and effort, in fact, nearly
everything could be repaired
and set to making music again.

A Cool Walk and a Hot Bath

T here were still a few leaves left on the trees, but not many.

I looked up from my spot on the gravel path at a lingering clump of oak leaves still hanging from a branch, held high against the gray sky. They were bright orange, and I imagined them holding on and making a pact to stay a bit longer, to last a few days more. I looked around through the trunks of the trees: frost lingered there, and the rising winds were pushing piles of dry brown pine needles and fallen leaves into clumps against roots and stumps. I drew a deep breath into my lungs and smelled less of the spicy smoky smell of autumn and more of the cool clean smell of the coming winter. Snow was coming, but I smiled up at the stubborn leaves; there was still a bit of time.

I pulled my hat a little lower around my ears and turned my face into the wind; it was cool but not sharp and made me feel awake. The path turned ahead of me to move beside a creek and I turned with it, watching water slip over mossy stones and pool in slow-turning eddies. In the spring I'd watched frogs from this spot, as they hid in the thick grass of the banks or floated with slow-blinking eyes just above the waterline. Ahead of me the creek picked up and spread and moved faster; I stopped at an old bridge and leaned over the railing, looking down at the water rushing past beneath me.

The wind was pushing me home now, and I tucked my hands into my pockets to warm them. Turning from the park I walked past a schoolyard where a few kids were kicking a ball and calling out shouts of excitement and jokes into the chilly air. They laughed and ran, red faces cooled in the wind, their jackets in a pile, forgotten and on their way to being lost. The wind blew harder and pushed a pile of fallen leaves up against a chain-link fence, a few stems catching and holding them there. "I'm going, I'm going," I told the wind.

Turning onto my street, I heard the muffled friendly bark of dogs in neighbors' houses, welcoming me back. I saw one, nose steaming against the window, happily shifting weight from paw to paw, and I called out to him and waved, and he barked back. A lot of comfort comes from just saying to a friend, "I see you." I turned to my own front porch and spotted a small package propped against the front door, smiled at my name on the label.

The warmth and the smell of home surrounded me as I hung up my coat and carried my paper-wrapped treasure to the kitchen table. Inside I found sweet-smelling soaps, salts, and a pretty bottle of bubble bath. They were tied in ribbons and wrapped in tissue, a gift. The fact that I'd sent this particular gift to myself made it no less sweet. *And my timing is perfect*, I thought. *A hot bath is just the thing*.

My tub is a big slipper tub, freestanding under a window in my bathroom, and as the water ran and began to steam, I cracked the window just a bit and let the cool fresh air mix with the steam. I trickled in the bubble bath and adjusted the water for the perfect temperature. Baths

212 · KATHRYN NICOLAI

were serious business to me and I planned accordingly; sometimes I had a glass of wine to sip or a bowl of apple slices to munch while I soaked; sometimes I clipped my hair up and painted on a face mask and pretended to be one of those people who know what to do with all the products that had sat for years under my sink. Today I wanted a tall bottle of mineral water, a glass full of ice, some music, and my book.

When my bath was ready, I set out a fresh fluffy towel on the radiator beside the tub to warm while I soaked, and I slipped one foot at a time into the water and lowered myself in. There's always that first rush of heat that makes me go still for a few moments. It pushes leftover thoughts out of my head and leaves me with the pure sensory delight of floating and heat. Minutes passed; I sipped my fizzy water, propped my heels on the edge of the tub, and watched steam rise from my skin. I read a few pages. I put my book down and listened to the music. I slid down into the water and reminded myself of the frogs blinking in the creek. Outside my window, the wind was still blowing; those kids from the park were probably coming through their front doors about now, smelling dinner and hungry for it. The neighbors' dogs were curled up on sofas or looking out of windows waiting to bark hello.

We were all tucked into our various nests and ready for the winter. Snow was coming; a few more weeks and we'd wake up one morning to a white crystallized landscape. I looked forward to a winter of long hot baths, to watching the snow fall from inside my cozy nest. I leaned my head back to rest against the edge of the tub and let my eyes close and the heat soothe my system. It was good to be so quiet.

Sweet dreams.

BATH-TIME RITUALS

. · . . ·

When my mother came home at the end of the day, she'd stand at a little cabinet tucked into a niche in the entryway and slowly slide the rings from her fingers, then unclasp her watch and place all the finery into a small ceramic bowl set there just for the purpose. She worked with her hands all day and they must have been sore. She'd massage her finger joints one by one and press the pad of her thumb into her palm, rubbing out the ache. Then she'd slide her wedding band back on, leaving the rest in the bowl to wait for her till tomorrow. She was quiet while she did this, slowly attending to her hands, and when she had finished, she'd let out a small sigh and step into the heart of the house and join us in the listening to and telling of the stories of the day.

Someone explained to me years ago that when rituals are blindly followed, they aren't of much use, but when they have a bit of meaning tied into them and when you think about that meaning while performing them, they can become tools. Tools that can help you turn the page on a moment, celebrate, treasure, or any number of useful human actions. When I learned that, I thought of my mother and her evening habit and the bowl on the cabinet. It had been a ritual of her own devising, a way to care for herself at the end of the workday and to shift from the world of traffic and deadlines to a world of her own with her family and home.

Here is a simple ritual for caring for yourself by taking a hot bath. You'll need the following:

A clean bathtub
Epsom salts or bubble bath, if you enjoy them
A candle
Matches or a lighter
A clean fluffy bath towel and washcloth

Every part of taking a bath takes time, so this is a ritual for slowing down. Sometimes rushing is contagious; we rush when don't mean to simply because the pace of the world around us is fast. Begin then by separating yourself from the world and its haste. Outside of your bathroom, find a place to switch off and set down things like your phone, your smartwatch, your tablet. Literally turn them off. These things are not coming with you into the bath and not even their vibrations or alerts are welcome.

Go into your bathroom and close the door. If you can, lock it. As you do, take a moment to simply notice that you are shutting the world out of your space. You are alone now. You might find you have been tensing your shoulders or jaw and now you can relax.

Turn on the water and adjust the taps until the water is exactly the temperature you enjoy. If you are using bubble bath or Epsom salts, add them now. Watch as the bubbles spread or the salt dissolves. You might find that your mind, so used to multitasking, wants to jump to another activity. It might be temporarily uncomfortable, but hold yourself there; don't become distracted. This is uni-tasking, and it can become very relaxing with practice.

When the bath is full, close the taps.

Light your candle. You can make an intention as you do so or just attend closely to the process of drawing the flame and lighting the wick.

Undress.

Set your towel within reach and your washcloth beside the tub.

As you lower yourself into the tub, pay attention to the feeling of the water on your skin. Lie back and just soak for ten minutes.

When you were bathed as a baby, you were carefully watched over. As you soap and wash yourself now, go slow, with the same kind of care. You have not stopped deserving care and attention.

When you exit the bath, pull the plug and stay in the bathroom as the tub drains. Wrap yourself in your towel or robe and rinse the bath with care. Leave it ready for the next bath. Snuff your candle and take a deep breath before you unlock the door.

You have cared for yourself; now nothing remains but to care for others.

A Rainy Day, Making Soup

I'd been out all day, umbrella open, going from shop to shop. I was finishing errands and racing through the rain. I'd bumped into an old friend along the way and we'd stopped into a café for a hot drink, settling into a couple of deep armchairs by a window and watching the rain coming down. It was only the early afternoon but the days were getting shorter, the skies were dark and low, and the bustle on the street was picking up as folks rushed to finish their errands, the instinct to nestle into our homes and hibernate getting stronger. We sipped our cooling drinks and chatted away for a while. I realized I'd been hurrying all day even though the deadlines I'd set myself were imaginary. I had time, and sitting with my friend, tasting the sweet hot chai in my cup, reminded me of that.

On our way back out into the afternoon, we made a date for lunch in a few days and gave each other a long squeeze. I notice that my oldest friends, when they wrap me in their arms for a hug, squeeze me fit to break my ribs. None of this leaning in with a light pat on the back stuff. It felt like a boost, like a spark deep inside that caught and lit me up with a soft glow.

Tucked under my umbrella, back in the rain, I smiled through my last few chores, and soon enough was turning the key in my front door and stepping into the warmth of home. I set down my bags, slipped my umbrella into the stand, and turned to lock the door. As I turned the bolt, I looked out at the rain, watched it running in heavy streams through gutters and downspouts, trailing down the sidewalks and coursing into the streets. I was home for the night and couldn't be happier about it. I smiled thinking of Mr. Rogers as I slipped out of my raincoat and into an old cardigan, then changed my wet shoes for fuzzy slippers.

I carried my purchases into the kitchen and set everything out on the counter. I felt that sticky habit of rushing creeping up on me again, and I stood still a second and took a big breath.

"You're home," I told myself. "You've got the whole evening laid out in front of you. Relax. Do what you like."

I looked around my kitchen. I always like to have a clean slate when I cook so I tidied away the few dishes and cups sitting in the sink, wiped down the counters, and lit the candle on my windowsill. *Much better*, I thought. *Now, shall I have a drink of something?* I started to fill the kettle for tea but remembered a bottle of something special in the fridge that I'd mixed up a few days before. I'd seen a recipe for a home-made kind of coffee cordial, made with whiskey and espresso, coconut milk, vanilla, and maple syrup. When I'd blended it up, I'd stirred some into a cup of coffee, which wasn't bad at all, but now I took a rocks glass from my cupboard, added a big ice cube, poured it straight from the fridge, and sipped it. It was creamy and a little sweet and the whiskey was smooth and had a golden maple flavor. I let it sit on my tongue for a few moments before swallowing it down and turning back to the counter of groceries.

It was the perfect night for a soup, and I set my biggest pot out on the stove. I chopped an onion, some garlic, carrots, and celery, and added them to my pot with a few spoonfuls of olive oil. As they warmed and sizzled in the oil, I opened a can of smoky crushed tomatoes, took some veggie broth from my cupboard, and chopped a big bunch of chard into strips. I always start a soup thinking I don't have enough to fill the pot but end up barely being able to get the lid on. The night before, I'd been looking through my cupboard and found a paper bag of bright red beans I'd bought at the farmers market at the end of the summer. The farmer had written in pencil across the bag, *Scarlett Runner, good for soup,* so I'd soaked them overnight in a bowl of water in my fridge. Now I drained and rinsed them, added them with the broth and tomatoes and brought it to a boil, then down to a simmer. As the flavors came together, I mixed up a quick cornbread and baked it in a cast iron pan in my oven.

I heard a key in the lock and another umbrella joining mine in the stand. "That smells amazing," I heard over stomping feet and the rustle of a raincoat. I smiled and rushed out to the entryway for my kiss. That light inside sparked again, and even in the chill of the anteroom with a cool nose pressed against mine, I was warm and rosy inside. "Dinner in a bit," I said. "Want a drink?"

"Yes, please. I'll have whatever you're having." I went back to the kitchen and stirred the soup, adding in the greens and turning off the heat. I cut up a couple lemons that I would squeeze in at the last moment. I am a firm believer that every single soup is improved by a squeeze of lemon right before it's eaten. I peeked at the bread, a lovely sweet steam escaping the oven as I did. Fifteen minutes, I guessed, and I could dish it all up. I heard an old movie click on and the sound of my sweetheart stretching out on the sofa. I poured a drink and carried it into the living room, set it down on the coffee table. I went back for mine and, stepping back into the room, heard a soft snore. I perched on the arm and raised my glass to my lips, thinking how good it was to be home together, quiet and relaxed on a dark rainy night.

Sweet dreams.

Homemade Irish Cream Cordial

. · . · .

MAKES 1 QUART

This lovely little concoction is excellent at the holidays. I often make up a batch before Thanksgiving and dole it out as friends stop by through the season, but it also makes a nice treat on any old day of the week. Make it as a gift for friends and neighbors or serve it with Christmas brunch.

1 can (13.5 ounces) full-fat coconut milk

2 tablespoons pure maple syrup, more to taste

1 tablespoon cocoa powder

1 teaspoon pure vanilla extract

2 shots of espresso or 1/4 cup strong coffee

1 cup Irish whiskey, such as Jameson

Add the coconut milk, maple syrup, cocoa powder, vanilla, and espresso to a blender. Blend on high for at least one minute, until the mixture comes together and is smooth and frothy.

Add the whiskey. Blend on high until combined. Taste for sweetness and feel free to add more maple syrup, if desired.

Enjoy over ice or stir an ounce or two into a cup of hot coffee. Store the cordial in an airtight container in the fridge for up to one month. If it separates, give it a good long shake or pop it back in the blender for a quick whizz before serving.

Outside at Night, with My Dog

I heard the soft pad of my dog's paws as he stopped beside the bed.

My ears were programmed to him by now. I heard when he sighed in the night or turned over in his bed. And when he got up to stand quietly beside me, I heard that too. He was an old boy, his muzzle gray and his gait slow and careful. Our walks had gotten a bit shorter, but today, he'd seen a squirrel racing along the sidewalk and had suddenly found a bit of young-dog energy in his limbs. He'd pulled me, chasing down the path. Thankfully, he hadn't caught it, but he liked the chase, barking as the squirrel ran up a tree and teased him, chittering away in the language of small animals who know how quick they are. I patted his head and told him he'd tried his best, and shouldn't we be getting on to the park?

I reached out now to rest my hand on him and swung my feet to the floor, sleepy but understanding. As he had gotten older he sometimes needed to go out in the middle of the night. I didn't mind at all. I wrapped my robe around me and pushed my feet into slippers, and we padded down the stairs and out to the backyard. Most times I'd just let him out and back in a few minutes later, but something about the way the air smelled as I opened the door pulled me out with him. It was pitch black, deep night, around 3:00 a.m. I guessed, and we were in those weeks when the weather played back and forth between autumn and winter. The cold air opened my eyes, and I turned them upward to see a clear sky lit by stars and a moon a little past half full. Waxing gibbous, I thought.

After my dog had come back to my side, we both stood very still and just listened. Summer nights have buzzing bugs, croaking frogs, and a sort of sourceless hum that comes from nowhere in particular but is simply present in the air. Maybe it is the fecundity of growing, surging plants or just the buzz of liveliness that is left over from a day in the sun, but it is undoubtedly noisy. There is a particular sound that you can hear only in the middle of the night in the near winter: a shocking quiet. There were no cars driving past, there were no animals up and about besides us, and there was only the faintest sound of a very light wind moving through the empty branches high above us. The land was sleeping, her creatures curled in dens, settling in for the new season. Bulbs were deep under mulch and dirt, only dreaming now of the bright pinks and purples and yellows they would unfold into in the spring.

We stood a moment more, and I let the cold air nip at my fingers and move over the back of my neck knowing that I'd be back in my warm bed soon. I took a few very deep breaths, and under the spicy scent of dry leaves there was something clean and clear in the air. I thought it might be snow. These clear skies could be thick with clouds tomorrow, and if we got up again in the middle of the night, as we probably would, we could be standing under the first falling flakes of the season.

I bent down and planted a slow kiss on the top of my old boy's head and we turned and went back inside. He stopped for a drink of water. I

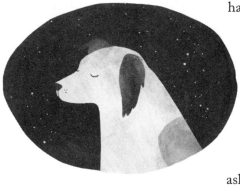

had one too, and then we slowly took the stairs back up to bed. He turned a few times and settled onto his big soft cushion. I spread his blanket over him and tucked it around his back. He'd be asleep in seconds. We should all learn this from dogs: they can go from completely awake to deeply asleep in moments and reverse it just as easily.

I slipped off my robe and slippers and pulled back the heavy quilt on my bed. I slid down into the sheets and smoothed the quilt over me. I felt the chill go out of my body by degrees until even the tips of my toes were warm again. I thought of the changing season, of the very quiet wind outside and how grateful I was that my dog had taken me out into it. This is a gift our friends give us: they take us places we wouldn't go on our own and show us things we'd have otherwise missed.

I took a slow breath and turned onto one side, tugging the quilt up over my shoulder. I felt myself drifting toward sleep. I'd pull some of today into my dreams as I nodded off. The squirrel flicking her tail high in the tree. The pull on the leash as my dog had suddenly wanted to run. The waxing moon and the sleeping land. The possibility of snow.

Yes, I was likely to be awakened again tomorrow night and many nights after that but I was happy for it.

Sweet dreams.

This is a gift our friends

give us: they take us places

we wouldn't go on our own

and show us things we'd

have otherwise missed.

The Day after Thanksgiving

Some people rush out on the day after Thanksgiving to mob the stores at four in the morning and shop till they drop, but I've never felt the slightest desire to join them.

In fact, I think the day after Thanksgiving is the perfect day to lie in bed for a long time, sip coffee, and think about which kind of pie you should have for breakfast. So that's what I was doing. I was on my second cup, swaddled deep in my pillows and comforter, while the rest of the house slept late. I was half reading a book and half remembering dinner the night before and smiling at the memories.

Our Thanksgiving is a sweet mix of family and a few friends so dear and long held that they might as well be family. It starts early, in the afternoon, as cars pull up and the doorbell rings. Casserole dishes carefully bundled in carriers get passed from hand to hand, drinks are poured, and groups form around dishes of nuts and trays of olives and pickles. Everyone helps out, stirring and tasting and laying the table, and finally we all sit down and raise our glasses to each other and to the year that's passed and to all that we have. Then the food and passing plates and laughing and refilling glasses and declarations about not being able to eat any more—and then, eating a bit more. There's always that lull after the meal, some needing to stretch out and maybe catch a little nap, the younger ones needing to blow off some steam and bundling up to play football outside, others happy to chatter and gossip while they clean and pack up leftovers and brew pots of coffee to go with the pies.

That brought me back to the question at hand. What kind of pie should I have for breakfast? I padded down to the kitchen, blessedly cleaned by the group effort the night before, and considered my options. Pumpkin. Apple. Pecan. That was tough. I had been known to choose the sampler option in the past, but today, I knew down deep the answer was pumpkin.

I cut myself a large wedge and poured another cup of coffee from the pot. I'd tried something new this year and whipped chilled coconut milk from the can into a creamy sweet topping. Some went onto the pie and some in my coffee. As I ate and sipped, I slid around in my socks and peered out through the windows. No snow yet, but the leaves had a crunchy hard frost on them and the air looked cold through the sunlight. I saw a bird, a bright red northern cardinal with a black face and red beak, at the feeder; in a branch beside him sat a silvery gray tufted titmouse, with a patch of blush peach on his side and belly. They ate well from our feeders but also pecked around at the shrubs and trees, finding a few leftover berries.

That made me think of the bowl of washed cranberries, ready in the fridge, that I'd forgotten to do anything with the day before. I clicked my tongue; oh well, nobody really eats the cranberries anyway. I'd string them instead, with popcorn, for the Christmas tree. Perfect.

To my pajamas and socks ensemble, I added an old green cardigan, buttoning it up as I headed to the closet to find my sewing needles and thread. They weren't really mine; I'd inherited an old case of supplies from an aunt who was a keen seamstress. When her eyes had gotten a bit too bad to keep working, she'd passed it to me, hoping I might take up the hobby. I hadn't, but I loved her case and took a moment to set it out on a table and go through some of her things. She had a fine pair of long silver scissors (I remembered as a child being told they couldn't be borrowed for any purpose other than sewing); an old red pin cushion that was fashioned liked a tomato but with a tiny strawberry hanging from it, still pricked with her needles and pins; and a glass jam jar full of buttons. I poured some out into my hand and poked through them, wondering what dress or suit jacket or fancy heeled shoe they'd come from. I selected some strong thread and the pin cushion with needles and packed up the rest and put it away.

I took out my bowl of cranberries and brought out the popcorn pan from the cupboard. I added oil and dropped in just three kernels of corn and put it on the stove.

(Listen, I'm about to tell you a secret about popcorn: wait for those three kernels to pop and once all three have, add the rest, and you'll pop everything in the pot by the time you're done without burning. I don't know how it works, but it does.)

I guessed that the smell of fresh popcorn and hot coffee would mean I would have company soon, and that sounded fine to me. I poured the popcorn into a huge bowl and salted it. I set myself up on the sofa with a long string of black thread, a needle, the popcorn and cranberries, and a bowl to catch the strung garland. I ate a piece and strung a piece and worked like that for a while, till I heard shuffling slippers on the stairs and a cup being filled in the kitchen.

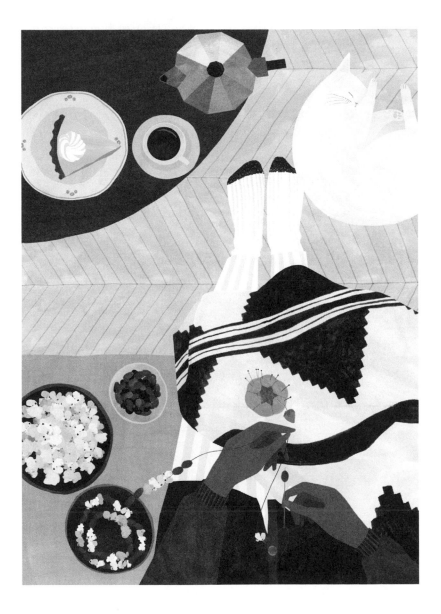

Sleepy eyes watched me over the rim as I threaded the berries and corn. "Where's the holiday music? And we should have a fire."

I smiled, knowing we had the whole day to do more of this.

"Yes, please," I said.

Sweet dreams.

Bustle in the City

From the frosty window of my little apartment I could see through the streets of downtown into the park, where the big city Christmas tree was being strung with lights.

It had come in on a long flatbed truck this morning, and since then, clusters of people bundled in coats had busied themselves around it. It had taken a while and some yelling and frantic arm waving from the people in charge, but now it stood straight and tall in the middle of the park, and in a few hours, it would be lit for the first time this season.

I stepped back from the window and looked around at my own snug space, which I'd just finished decorating. Strings of colored fairy lights circled around the windows and stretched across the bricks and beams of the old apartment. My little tree, set up on a table by the window, with just lights and some paper ornaments I'd cut myself, blinked merrily. I knew my neighbor and her little girl in the apartment across the street would be able to see it from their window, and I liked that. I could see their menorah from where I stood and had been invited to light the first candle of the nine with them a few nights ago. We'd played games and shared a big meal and promised to go skating in a few weeks.

I took a last sip from my cup of cinnamon coffee and set it in the sink. I was meeting some friends in the park for the tree lighting, but first I had a bit of shopping to do. I pulled on my boots, wrapped my coat and scarf tight around me, found the mittens I'd somehow not lost yet, and headed out from my apartment, on the third floor of an old brick building right in the center of the town. I took the stairs down to the street and stepped out into the afternoon air. It was cold and I filled my lungs, smelling the chilled clean scent of snow in the air and the fresh green pine scent of the tree that would be lit tonight.

On the street level of our building, we had a sweet little bookshop that I stopped into at least once a week. They were open late tonight, and I looked in through the shop front and watched a few people browsing and reading. They had a reading nook set right into the front window of the shop with a broad wooden bench and a curved canopy of walnut above it. A boy in his teens sat in it engrossed in a book about a starship and a mission to Mars. I saw the owner of the shop behind the register, and we waved at each other as I started to walk.

The streets were busy, people shopping, looking at the window displays, and bumping into friends on the corners. I had a favorite shop on the next street; they sold pretty stationery, funny old cards, and a strange collection of music, nice-smelling soaps, potted plants, and hand-knitted scarves. I had a feeling that the owner just randomly bought anything he liked and put it out without any sort of plan. Sometimes the best plan is no plan. I was looking for a card for a friend of mine who lived on the other side of the world. I didn't send many holiday cards but I wanted to send one to her. I liked thinking of her opening her mailbox and seeing my handwriting on the envelope and feeling like she was home. I thumbed through the cards and found one with a vintage illustration that reminded me of my little tree up in the window. I bought it and tucked it into my bag and stepped back out onto the streets. I stopped in a few more shops on my way to meet my friends; I bought a pair of earrings to send to my sister, a book about identifying native birds for a friend, and, on a whim, a jigsaw puzzle for the little girl across the street. I could hear music coming from the park; it was getting darker, and I made my way through the bustling crowds to the center of town.

I spotted my friends clustered around the front door of a coffee shop across from the park, and I called out to them. This was a yearly tradition, sometimes we got dinner, sometimes we sat in the pub all night, but always we watched the tree lighting and shared some holiday cheer. We were a big group and took over some seats and benches around a heater on the edge of the park. Someone had thought ahead and brought a thermos of hot chocolate and some paper cups. We passed it around and sent a few of our number out to the street vendors for popcorn and those hot candied nuts they tie into paper cones.

The square around us was filling with people: friends, shopkeepers, people I passed on the street every day, families with kids sitting on shoulders to get a good view of the tree. It was almost time. The band got a bit louder and the crowd turned its attention to the center of the square. Someone with an old microphone was speaking on a fuzzy far-off speaker, telling us what we already knew. The holidays were here. In the dark nights, there was also light, and coming together to share it was a good idea.

The drum rolled, the kids clapped and stomped in a fever of

anticipation. There was a moment of quiet all over the city, and then the lights came on. A tower of a tree stood, lit in her glory in our park, and we all clapped and whistled our approval.

Not long after, we called it a night. We squeezed hands and hugged and pressed chilled cheek to chilled cheek and said happy holidays and be safe and sleep tight. The streets were looped with strings of lights, and I took my time, walking back to my flat, looking in the shop windows and smelling the good smells of the vendors and cold night air along the way.

I liked my life. I liked to be out in the bustle of the city, out with my friends, busy and merry on a December night, but I also liked the quiet solitude of my little apartment. The stillness, the simple decorations I'd set up, the sound of the old radiators hissing with steam. The bookshop was closed now, the streets were quieting, and just as I turned to go in, a few silent flakes floated down and I caught them in the palm of my mittened hand. I smiled up at the streetlights showing a pattern of fluffy flakes coming down.

I couldn't wait to watch them from my favorite window upstairs, curled on my chair with a blanket pulled around me. I turned the key and tucked myself in for the night.

Sweet dreams.

The holidays were here.

In the dark nights, there was

also light, and coming

together to share it was

a good idea.

HANDMADE PAPER ORNAMENTS

. · . · .

I've been making these simple hand-cut ornaments for years. Sometimes I make them very large, from colored cardstock, and other times I make them from origami paper, which comes in many beautiful colors. They are a great craft to make with young children because they are so simple and quick. You can nestle them into the boughs of a Christmas tree, tuck them into the greenery on your mantel or hang them from thread at your window.

12 sheets of 6-x-6-inch origami paper
     in a range of colors
Pencil
Good sharp scissors
A spool of thread or dental floss, for
     hanging
Glue and glitter

Fold a sheet of origami paper in half. Use your pencil to trace out a shape like the one pictured. Once you've made a few of these you may want to try changing the shape a bit. You could make your ornament rounder at the bottom or skinnier or boxy. There's no way to do it wrong, so just play around.

Cut all the way around the shape. You can cut just inside of the pencil line so you don't see it on the finished piece, or you can erase the lines later if you like. Then cut along the three lines in the middle. Notice that those lines don't go all the way through the shape; if you cut too far, you'll end up with an ornament in pieces. Just cut in an inch or so. Cut out the small diamond-shaped notch in the top of the ornament if you'd like to hang it.

Open up the ornament. The slits in the middle can help give it more shape. Push the strip under the first cut back and re-crease it along the original fold. Draw the next strip forward and re-crease it. Push the last strip back and re-crease one more time.

You can cut string or floss to thread through the top notch and hang your ornaments or just place them wherever you like. You can also use some glue to stick some glitter around the edges to make them shine.

Getting the Tree

There was a little bistro on a corner, a few blocks from our house.

It was a long, narrow place, with deep booths and low lights and a bar stretched against one wall. They'd strung some twinkle lights around the sills of the big street-side windows, and each table had a candle or two glowing in glass jars. We were headed out to get our Christmas tree, but first we needed a bite and drink. We were lucky and got the last booth, in a cozy corner where we could lean back and watch the people strolling on the streets and cars with trees strapped to their roofs driving by.

Even though it was a week past, we were still a little full from Thanksgiving, so we just asked for some snacks and two glasses of champagne. The waiter delivered a broad tray of nibbles for us. It held toasted nuts seasoned with rosemary and orange rind, still warm from the pan. A basket of bread, soft on the inside but with a good crust around it, a deep dish of olive oil speckled with dark balsamic vinegar and scattered with herbs, a tiny dish of braised artichokes and mushrooms, and some fat green olives. He set down the champagne, and beside it a small plate of red raspberries. We smiled our thanks and lifted our glasses to each other and the merry day that lay ahead. I took a sip from my glass and let it fizz on my tongue for a moment, looking out to the street as the first few flakes started to fall. *Bubbles*, I thought, *go very well with snowflakes.*

We took our time, munching and sipping our way through the meal. We planned a bit, talked about the things we wanted to do before the season was over: ice skating, a holiday party, an old Christmas movie that was showing at the theater. And we sat quiet for a bit, just enjoying the snowfall and the flavors. What a gift it is to have someone that you can be quiet with, that you can share a simple moment of enjoyment with. I didn't take it for granted. I said a silent thank-you deep in my heart and let myself feel the warm, contented glow that my good luck has brought me.

When we'd paid our bill and wound our scarves around our heads, re-mittened and re-hatted, we stepped out into the falling snow and stood a moment to let it catch on our faces and to smell the good cold scent of the winter. We climbed into our car and headed out to the tree farm.

When I was a child, my folks, bless them, bundled us up every year and took us out to cut our own tree. There was a hayride and a long walk through snowy fields and quite a bit of family deliberation about which tree felt just right to each of us. As an adult I appreciate the effort that went into that day, and I smile looking back at the memories and the leftover feeling of childlike excitement that still lingers around them.

A few years back, we'd found a place that had a good stock of fresh trees and a sweet little shop in an old farmhouse that sold glass ornaments and hot cider and had a big crackling fire in the hearth that made me quite happy to forgo cutting our tree ourselves.

We pulled into the snowy lot and parked along a row of leaning trees ready for their homes. There are some things you are never too old for, and the happy excitement of a Christmas tree is one of them. "Come on, love," I said, clapping my mittened hands together. "Let's find our tree."

We walked through the fresh falling snow and started to consider the options. We like a tall Charlie Brown tree, a little spindly and with big gaps to hang our favorite ornaments, but they are hard to find. We recognized a man bundled up in overalls, eyes bright in the cold, as the same one who'd helped us the year before, and he waved us over. He said he had just the tree for us, that he'd remembered us and when he'd seen a tall, spare, gangly tree in his field, he'd cut it hoping we'd be back. And here we were. I thanked him for his kindness in remembering us and left him to the work of hoisting it up onto the car and securing it with loops of strong brown twine while I slipped into the farmhouse for a couple cups of something warm.

Really, more than the hot drink, I wanted a chance to poke around the shop and pet the kitty who lived there. It was wonderfully warm inside and made me feel how cold I'd gotten. I stopped in front of their fire for a few moments and stretched my fingers toward the warmth in the grate. The little house was strung with lights and smelled of the fresh pine boughs tucked onto every spare shelf. I ordered a hot cocoa and a cider, and pointing through the window to the kind man who was wrestling our tree up onto the roof of our car, I asked, "What does he like to drink?"

"Oh, he'd probably like a coffee," the lady behind the counter told me.

"Then a coffee too, please."

"I know how he likes it, black with two sugars," she said with a wink.

As she took my few dollars and busied herself with my order, I heard a low meow from my ankles and looked down to see their spotted kitty winding through my legs. I squatted down, petted her head, and chatted with her a moment. She was soft with a big friendly belly, and when she tired of me, she strutted off to find someone else to talk to. I took the drinks outside and handed them out, saying thank you and happy holidays and see you next year, and we climbed in our car and started for home.

Sweet dreams.

Snowed In

The day before, they'd said it would snow all night and through the next day.

They said that the drifts would pile up into our doorways and alleyways, in our fields and intersections, and that we had all better stay safe in our houses. We agreed. Across the village, through the county, we agreed. Today, we were all snowed in.

I lay in my bed, in the muffled quiet of the early morning, thinking about the snow, settled like a thick blanket on the ground, on the bare limbs of trees, on the roof above my head, and on every surface it could find. I didn't move yet, just felt my limbs relaxed and warm under the comforter and thought how good it is to know that you have a snow day and how it is even better to have known it the night before. I'd slept deep and woke without remembering my dreams, feeling like I had a clean slate for the day. I slipped my feet into the waiting slippers beside my bed, pulled a long, thick sweater over my shoulders, and stepped to the window. I pulled back the curtain slowly and enjoyed the small spark of anticipation in my belly as I looked out at the covered land.

I grew up with snow; I've seen this a thousand times. I've

experienced this same moment since I was a child—the morning after a heavy snowfall, standing in pajamas with my nose pressed against a cold windowpane—but every time, I'm still amazed. The morning light was thin and threw long shadows over the drifts, caught the still-falling flakes in their airy descent and showed the crisp, unbroken surface of snow sloping through the land around my old farmhouse. I took a moment there, just watching the snow fall, my arms wrapped around me against the chill of the window, and enjoyed the gift of a day blocked off by Mother Nature.

As a child, snow days were about excitement and rushing from the snow and the sled to the warm kitchen for cups of cocoa and back out again. As an adult, they are a relief. You're forced to relax, and no one could reasonably expect anything from you for the day. And in a busy world that sometimes moves too fast, that respite is good medicine.

I'd stocked up the day before, and my kitchen was full of all the snow-day necessities: a pound of fresh coffee beans, a long loaf of bread for sandwiches and toast, a bakery bag full of scones and muffins, a sack of winter oranges and grapefruits. My fridge held a jug of fresh juice and plenty of green vegetables, and in my pantry I had neat rows of home-canned tomatoes and pickles, jars of beans, sacks of rice, and packages of crackers and pastas. I looked out the kitchen window and said to the falling snow, "Keep coming down; I've enough for a few weeks."

I started brewing some coffee, poked around the muffins, broke off a corner of one and nibbled it. If you're going to do it, I thought, might as well do it right, and pulled the waffle iron out of a cupboard. After all, this was part of the joy of a snow day, having time to do the things you usually didn't and no reason at all not to. I poured a cup of coffee, pulled some ingredients from shelves and started mixing and whisking and heating the iron. I set a place for myself at the kitchen table with my favorite chipped plate, a napkin, and a fork.

I had a flash of memory, something my aunt had done when we were young. She had a special plate in her cupboard, it was painted gold in an old pattern and matched nothing else, and if you'd done well on a test, or if it was your birthday, or if you'd had a bad day and just needed to feel special and cared for, she set it at your place. When you sat down, you'd sit a bit taller, feel her warm hand on your shoulder. Dinner was sweeter.

The memory warmed me through as I ladled batter into the hot iron, and I smiled as it sizzled and scented the air. With pancakes and waffles, it's always the rule of three. Undercook the first one, burn the second one, and the third is perfect. Once I had a plateful, I sat with a fresh cup of coffee and a warmed jug of maple syrup and watched the snow come down as I ate. I peeled an orange and ate the segments slowly between sips. I set aside the peel, thinking that I might add it to a simmer pot later, with cinnamon sticks and vanilla and a few cloves. I'd let it simmer away all day to fill the house with its sweet scent and soften the dry air with its steam. I rinsed my plate and tidied up the kitchen and walked from window to window looking out.

I'd brought in firewood the night before and had the grate filled and ready to light. I struck a long match and held it to the paper and kindling, watching it take and burn. I laid in a few bigger pieces and squatted on the hearth for a few moments till my face and fingers were warmed through. The wind was blowing now, and I watched as little swirling spirals of snow appeared and diminished in the air. Maybe later I'd bundle up and take a long tromp through the fields and woods, then reward myself with a cup of something hot; but for now I didn't intend to leave my cozy spot. I could see myself spreading a jigsaw puzzle over the table and working away at it while a movie played in the background, or reading for hours, or lying in a hot bath till my fingers turned pruney. But first, full from breakfast and warm in front of the fire, I stretched out onto the sofa, pulled a long blanket over my legs, and felt like the best idea was probably to close my eyes, listen to the crackle of the logs, and take a long winter's nap.

Sweet dreams.

A Simmer Pot Recipe for Each Season

. . . . .

Simmer pots can add moisture to and lightly scent the air in your home. I find them particularly helpful during the winter when the air is dry, especially when we have frequent fires in our fireplace. But any time of year is a good time to make up a simmer pot. Often if I have one going when a friend stops by, they are surprised by how good the contents smell, and for those who find candles and other room fresheners irritating to the lungs, this method can be a soothing alternative.

Start by bringing a large soup pot full of water to a slow simmer on your stove. While you should never leave a simmering pot completely unattended, this can safely simmer for hours without going dry. Peek at it now and then, and if the water dips below 5 inches from the bottom, top it up. Add the following, depending on the season:

SPRING

Handful of dried lavender buds

A few sprigs of rosemary

2 teaspoons lemon extract

A few star anise pods

SUMMER

Peel from 2 large oranges

1 teaspoon pure vanilla extract

1 tablespoon cardamom seeds

FALL

2 cinnamon sticks

2 pine cones

1 red apple, sliced

1 teaspoon pumpkin pie spice

WINTER

1 orange, sliced

3 to 4 small cuttings from a pine tree

12 whole cloves

A Night at the Theater

We'd seen the ad before Thanksgiving.

It was for a show at the big theater downtown, something lighthearted and maybe a little silly, with dancing and singing and a live orchestra, playing through the whole month of December. We'd each read the ad separately and tore it out from our respective papers to show the other. We laughed when we presented our scraps of paper over dinner one night. We don't usually go in for big musicals and tend to like the smaller intimate shows in the little black box theaters that we knew, but I guess, at the holidays, we both wanted to see something that made us smile and tap our toes along to the music. For me, maybe it was because the holidays made me feel like a kid again; when I was little, my family had always gone to a big show at the theater in the week or so before Christmas. We would get a bit dressed up, shiny shoes and good coats and a little purse that I'd put some precious objects into. Kids have a way of making treasures out of the everyday. I'd probably had some little trinket earned in school, a whistle or a piece of sea glass, a tiny pencil and notepad, a very small bottle of perfume likely found in my mother's drawer, and a ring of spare keys that I pretended to need. We'd be taken out for a meal and strongly encouraged not to mess up our good clothes too early in the evening. When we arrived at the theater, I'd goggle at the people in fancy suits and dresses in the lobby. The theater itself seemed enormous, like a cathedral. I'd stand and gape at the details in the archways and the murals painted across the ceiling, the lush red carpet and brass banisters and the long winding staircase leading up to the balcony.

My father would tuck my hand into his elbow and lead me up to our seats. I'd sit with my feet swinging a foot off the floor, a program clutched in my hand and the incredible excitement in my belly that comes from getting ready to see a live performance. When the lights dimmed and the conductor struck up the orchestra, I'd open my eyes as wide as they'd go and listen with all my might so as not to miss a note or a fast-stepping shuffle-ball-change or a joke. By the end of the night we'd be that mix of keyed up and worn out that happens so easily when you're little, and we'd be tucked into the car and driven home. Along the way we'd circle through the neighborhoods to look at the houses decked out in Christmas lights. I remember leaning my cheek against the cool window in the back seat, letting the lights reflect on my face and dreaming about putting on my own show of song and dance.

Thinking of all these memories, I bought us tickets.

On the night of the show I put on my favorite red dress. I still carried a purse with little treasures inside but now, except for the tiny pencil and notebook, they looked a bit different and included a lipstick in a daring shade of bright red, a change purse with a few coins, and a carefully kept paper fortune that had come out of a cookie on our first date. I dabbed a bit of perfume behind my ears and wound a silky scarf around my neck. What fun, to revisit a moment I'd loved as a child with the perspective of a grown-up.

Before the show started, we went to a favorite restaurant, bustling with the holiday crowd. Normally I'd prefer the quiet, but tonight everyone was so merry. I looked across the tables around us and saw so many people lifting their glasses in celebration, so many sincere smiles and sparkling eyes that I felt happy to be surrounded by fellow revelers. We toasted each other as we sipped and ate. Even though we'd had many holidays together, there were still things we didn't know about each other, so we shared some memories we'd somehow never shared before. I thought that it was lovely, really, to share your life with someone and, decades into the sharing, still be able to surprise each other.

The theater had an old-fashioned ticket window where I stopped to claim our tickets. I'd always liked that moment when they were pushed through the little gap under the window, into the brass tray.

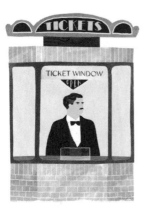

When I took them I smiled at the man behind the window and he smiled back.

The lobby was busy just as it had been in my memory and as my sweetheart's hand slipped into the crook of my elbow I stopped to watch a little boy staring up at the ceiling, his mouth open and his eyes wide.

We moved with the crowd, jostled a bit though we didn't mind. We found our seats and sat in excited anticipation as people streamed in. I peered down into the orchestra pit and saw musicians dressed in elegant black, ready with violas propped on their knees, or adjusting the reeds of their clarinets, or testing the slide on their trombones. The conductor was thoughtfully turning through the pages, one hand moving in the secret language of tempos and notation, skimming one more time through the score before the curtain was raised.

I thought of the actors in dressing rooms, applying the last of their makeup, the backstage crew checking props and cues. We were all coming together to do something and see something spectacular. That's often when humans are at our best, when we unite to create. The lights began to dim, the conductor raised her baton, and all of us seated there turned our collective attention to the stage.

Sweet dreams.

Christmas Eve

'd woken up with a feeling of electric excitement—that something was happening. Something good.

I lay still for a few moments and then smiled into my pillow. It was Christmas Eve. A day I loved and waited for all year. I sat up slowly in the darkness. I could hear the soft, slow breaths of my sweetheart sleeping and, not wanting to interrupt the slumber, I slipped out of bed. My dog was lying across the foot of the bed and she opened one brown eye to look at me. I squatted down beside her and whispered in her ear, "It's Christmas Eve." She listened, and I scratched her neck and leaned in to kiss the soft broad space between her eyebrows. As I moved to the door she jumped down and followed me out; we closed the bedroom door behind us and tiptoed toward our morning routine.

As the kettle boiled, I watched my dog through the kitchen window as she inspected the backyard and weaved through the trees strung with lights, a few birds waking and hopping through the branches above her. I opened my front door just to see the houses still lit up from the night before, strings of lights outlining the roof peaks, woven around windows and circling tree trunks and branches. I heard the whistling kettle and went back in to fill my cup, and I found my dog waiting at the back door. I went to turn on the Christmas tree lights and set myself up on the couch. She sidled up next to me and lay with her head on my lap. I spread a blanket over us. The house was quiet and dark but for the glow of the tree. I laid my hand into the thick fur of her back as we sat and I sipped from my cup.

I'd had a dog years ago who didn't have much use for snuggling and affection. She was happy to lie in her own bed and just be in the room with me, but once a day or so, she would amble up to me and press her warm forehead against my thigh. I'd rub the back of her neck and after a moment she'd walk away and get back to whatever dog business occupied her time. Now, on the sofa with this little girl, I sat and said a silent thank-you to every dog everywhere for their friendship. I had a sneaking suspicion, one that grew stronger as I grew older, that the point of everything is just to make friends, just to share moments, to be there with whoever was there and to pay attention to all of it.

That's what I intended to make today about. We were having a little party, some food and music, a fire in the fireplace. I'd dusted off the piano and hoped someone would play a few songs. I felt a warmth spreading in my chest, grateful that faithful friends who were dear to us would gather near to us once more.

I'd spent the day before happily in the kitchen—my apron dusty with flour and powdered sugar, and the counters filling with baked treats: glossy golden braided breads, star-shaped cookies spread with frosting and dotted with tiny silver balls, and pastry cookies rolled with walnuts and cinnamon and glazed with apricot jam. I'd even baked a few homemade dog biscuits for Santa Paws to deliver to our little pooch.

I'd also made trays of finger foods, little tempting tarts filled with sun-dried tomatoes and pine nuts and caramelized onions. I'd serve bowls of roasted brussels sprouts, their outer leaves dark brown, crisp, and salty, and cold plates of dips and seasoned rice rolled into grape leaves. Some people dread being in the kitchen all day, but for me, especially at this time of year, it is merry work. I'd turned on an old favorite Christmas movie, black-and-white, one I'd seen a hundred times, and let it play while I worked my way through the dishes. When everything was done and the kitchen was set back to rights, I stepped back and sighed with satisfaction. My friends and family would be well fed. My home would be a haven for the people I loved. They would feel safe and relaxed and cared for, and that was just about my favorite thing.

Back on the couch, my dog softly snoring beside me, I thought through the rest of the day. There was time for a walk outside together, and time for me to hole up somewhere and wrap a few gifts. We could sample all the treats I'd made, catch each other under the mistletoe, and as evening darkness came on we would don our gay apparel, light the fire and the candles, lay out the trays of food, open the bottles of wine, and wait for our friends to come trekking up the driveway.

As a little girl watching old Christmas movies from the couch, I'd expected my grown-up holidays to be full of train trips through snowy countrysides and nights out in swanky cocktail clubs. I thought people might suddenly break out into tap dances in ski chalets, or at least that there would be . . . I guess . . . Muppets? As an actual adult, my holidays have been infinitely simpler: just a time to do some favorite things, to be closer to the people I called family, to wonder at the beauty of fresh snow or a lighted Christmas tree through a stranger's window. And to sit, with a hot cup of something lovely, on the couch with my dog, and be grateful for another year together.

Sweet dreams.

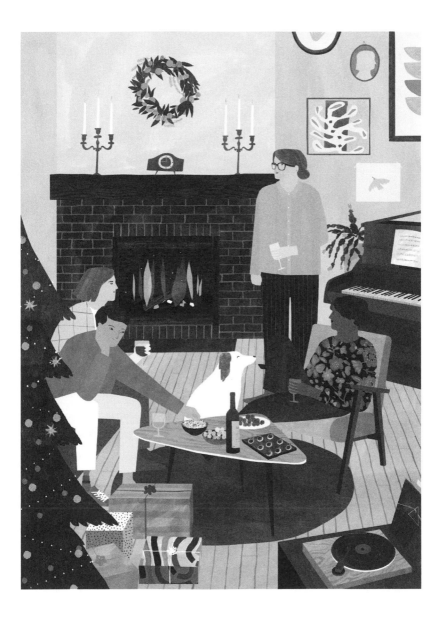

I had a sneaking suspicion,

one that grew stronger as

I grew older, that the point of

everything is just to make

friends, just to share moments,

to be there with whoever was

there and to pay attention

to all of it.

MEDITATION FOR A BUSY HOLIDAY

. · . · .

Find someplace away from others, someplace quiet where you can sit or lie down and be alone for a few minutes.

Settle your body with care in any posture that feels good. Close your eyes and take a deep breath in through your nose and sigh it out through your mouth. Let your lips touch back together and breathe naturally through your nose. Instead of demanding that your mind switch immediately to the present moment, allow your thoughts to slowly lose momentum.

Give yourself a moment to feel whatever there is to feel. Maybe there is a lot to do and you feel rushed. Maybe there are memories and traditions on your mind and you feel pressured or worried. Maybe there are people coming or already here and you feel that strange combination of excited and anxious that only family can evoke. Maybe you are at ease, relaxed and just looking to connect. However you feel is how you feel. As you connect to your present state of mind and emotions, look for the corresponding sensations in your body. Every emotion creates a physical sensation, and being able to read those sensations creates an early warning system as well as an awful lot of personal insight.

You'll notice that when you give your emotions your full

attention, when you listen to them deeply without trying to change them, they settle. I think of it sometimes like when you are meeting a friend in a restaurant. When you come in the door and they see you, they stick their arm straight in the air and wave frantically, but as soon as you make eye contact, they put their arm down and relax. They have been seen; they are calmer. So it is with the pressing emotions in our hearts and minds. They need to be seen and felt, and once they are, they often diminish.

Once the waves inside you have softened into ripples, turn your attention to the small space under the tip of your nose and above the base of your upper lip. Notice your breath moving in and out. When the mind wanders, acknowledge where it has gone. You don't have to pretend that your thoughts aren't there. See them. Feel them. Then come back to that small ridge in your upper lip and notice the breath.

When you are ready to rejoin the festivities, take another deep breath in through your nose and out through your mouth. Good.

Acknowledgments

First, I thank my lovely wife, Jacqui, who, from the moment I first had the idea for *Nothing Much Happens*, encouraged and supported me. She has never been surprised by any success that this project has achieved, having believed so completely in me and in what I set out to do. Being in love with her inspires a thousand grateful thoughts and happy possibilities every day, so when people ask me if I think I might at some point run out of sweet stories to tell, I can smile and confidently shake my head no. (Jacqui, I love you madly.)

Thank you to my parents. They taught me to love books and stories from my earliest years and then led me to believe that I was capable of just about anything I could imagine. When I was unsure, I trusted in their faith in me.

Thank you to my brother, Greg, a wonderful writer himself. When I called with an idea for a book (not this one, another), worried that it might not believably fit into this world, he simply said, "Sister, every book takes place in an alternate universe. Write what you like." So I did.

Thank you to my editors and publishers who have all been kind, creative, patient, and supportive. They are helping me bring this special kind of comfort to so many, and that is the realization of the biggest dream of my life. Special thanks to Meg Leder and Laura Dosky of Penguin who helped this first-time author think bigger and more vibrantly about the world I am creating.

Thank you to my agent, Jackie Kaiser. From our very first phone call, she completely and intuitively understood what I was trying to create. She asked me questions that kept my writing mind whirring and buzzing with excited energy, and I can't wait to see what else we dream up together.

Thank you to Léa Le Pivert for her beautiful illustrations. I have no inner eye and couldn't offer much, besides my words, to the look of *Nothing Much Happens*. Léa made it so beautiful and inclusive and warm. I'll always be grateful.

Thank you to my friends at Curiouscast for helping me to spread stories through the podcast to so many.

Thank you to the man, the legend, Bob Wittersheim, who makes the podcast sound so lovely and is so generous with his time and talent.

Thank you to everyone who has patiently listened to me while I learned how to tell a story (podcast listeners, yoga students, friends).

Thank you to Mary Oliver for all of her words, her poetry, and her instructions for living. When I heard her say, "Pay attention. Be astonished. Tell about it." I felt like I had found my vocation.

Index of Coziness

Note: The page numbers below indicate the first page of each story that includes that item of coziness.